Stay HEALTHY FIT & FINE

— The Natural Way

Luis S.R. Vas & Anita S.R. Vas

PUSTAK MAHAL®

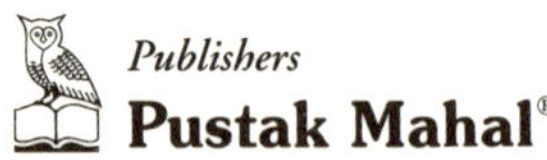

Publishers
Pustak Mahal®

Administrative office and sale centre
J-3/16 , Daryaganj, New Delhi-110002
☎ 23276539, 23272783, 23272784 • *Fax:* 011-23260518
E-mail: info@pustakmahal.com • *Website:* www.pustakmahal.com

Branches
Bengaluru: ☎ 080-22234025 • *Telefax:* 080-22240209
E-mail: pustak@airtelmail.in • pustak@sancharnet.in
Mumbai: ☎ 022-22010941, 022-22053387
E-mail: rapidex@bom5.vsnl.net.in
Patna: ☎ 0612-3294193 • *Telefax:* 0612-2302719
E-mail: rapidexptn@rediffmail.com

This book was earlier published under the title
"The Joy of Natural Living"

ISBN 978-81-223-0723-8

Edition: 2013

Printed at : **Sharma Printers, Delhi.**

Dedicated to

Heidi, Ulrich and Desiree,
Our Godchildren

CONTENTS

Introduction

We have been collecting research findings on subjects that fascinated us: health, psychology, body care, spirituality.... Over the years the material grew quite massive and we offered it to interested parties as a series of self-development audio cassette programmes. Eventually, we thought of presenting the material in a more permanent form, that is, print.

The present volume covers some of this material which, we trust, the reader will find useful. Research is a never ending process and is never final. Often, subsequent research contradicts previous findings. We present the findings in this book in the spirit of sharing information which we found useful. There is no substitute for testing its usefulness for yourself since, we believe, life itself is a series of experiments through which we learn new things all the time. Do not forget to consult your family doctor or a specialist before taking important decisions regarding your health.

A common theme runs through all the material gathered here. The more natural you are, the more joy you get out of life. Unfortunately, not only our environment, but also our own beings are being increasingly polluted by needless, often dangerous, accretions. We hope the reader will be able to regain some of his or her natural joy by experimenting with some of the advice presented here.

For example, psychologist Barry Long insists that "You are dissipating your energy through the personality, instead of using it to stay in your reality. The mask is kept on by energy going out. As you deny the projection of the personality, you conserve energy. When enough energy is retained, the mask collapses. It loses its independence and selfish existence. I'm going to show you where you're wasting this energy. Since you will then be conscious of it because you've seen it in your own experience, you'll begin to stop the leakage. You'll have more energy to address other wasteful mannerisms, attitudes and behaviour. Gradually you'll become more conscious, more responsible, more authentic. Your character will reveal itself and your personality will be less in control of your life. Anger arises because you are not getting your own way. I am going to mention several things to do or stop doing. They will conserve your energy. To begin with, it will be a challenge. As you get deeper into the process, you may become confused. The personality will always be trying to bamboozle you and make you give up. But "keep going." Long prescribes six exercises to "remind you and guide you. Your own undeniable experience that it's working will be the demonstration of the truth. You will notice that you are lighter, easier, more joyous. A new harmony will start pervading your whole life, within and without." The exercises are the following:

1. **Stop talking about the past.** Long points out that "the personality lives off the past and feeds off you telling your story. Each time you hear yourself indulging in talking about the past, stop. The more you practise, the easier it gets... There will be times when you have to refer to the past. However, to break the old habit, initially you must be extreme. The extremity is to not say anything that refers to the past. This includes what happened a minute ago, unless there's a purely practical reason for speaking, such as 'Did you post that letter?' By stopping talking about the past you will eventually stop thinking about the past. And that will be the beginning of the end of worry."
2. **Be true to the situation, not to your likes and dislikes.** Long gives the example that if you're employed to do a job, be true to what you're paid for, not to whether you like it or don't like it. "If you insist on reacting in dislike, be true to the situation and resign, because clearly, you won't be doing a good job."
3. **Beware of anger.** Anger, resentment, depression mean you are not facing life as it is. Anger indicates you are not getting your own way. When you get angry, stop and look at what practical steps you can take to remove the obstruction. If there is no practical way out you can think of, your desire is impractical at this time. To be honest you must face the fact and give up your wanting.

4. **Don't talk unless you've got something to say.** Your personality is constantly talking and in doing so it consumes enormous energy. This exercise is designed to enable you to talk less. By 'talking' Long refers to "talking about something, having a discussion, giving your opinions, speculating, rationalizing and repeating what you've heard." By doing this exercise, you learn the difference between talking and speaking. "Everyone talks about what the politicians should do. You can't talk about what the politicians should do unless you do something yourself towards righting the situation: write to the politicians, phone them or cast your vote. Then you'll be taking action and be able to speak from your own experience. Otherwise you're just a talker. Only action, or speaking what you live, is true."
5. **No more complaining and blaming.** Complaining and blaming other people for what happens to you is a major source of energy leakage. When you notice yourself doing this, stop. If it is your life, you are responsible for it. Otherwise, it's not your life and you're giving up responsibility by giving it to others. "To be responsible is to be responsible for everything that happens to you, unfolding as your life."
6. **Tackle habitual small talk.** The personality survives on habitual activity which is unconscious. Stop the conversational habit of using expressions like darling, honey, my love, and my dear when addressing your partner, friends or casual contacts, Long advises. If at all, use the person's correct name. To break the habit and make the situation conscious, also avoid common expressions like: 'What I mean is' and 'You know?' or any similar fill-in phrases. These are all unconscious habit-words of the personality, now become globally habitual. Don't say 'To be honest': it implies you're about to be dishonest, or that you're usually a liar. They are meaningless expressions and are actually the mask talking.

Long assures you that if you practise these exercises in your daily life over the next twelve months or so, you'll slowly separate yourself from the domination of the personality.

Long emphasises the joy within. "Life is to be enjoyed, to be made conscious by enjoying it. For joy is consciousness. When you enjoy anything you do, you are conscious. If you enjoy dancing, you're conscious while dancing. If you enjoy gardening, you're conscious while gardening. If you enjoy your work, you're conscious while working. Enjoy every moment of your life and you're living consciously as well as joyously. It's as simple as that. Joy or consciousness is your natural state. It's always there. It's like the sun that is always shining above the shadow of the earth and clouds. Stop living in your own shadow, and the sun, the joy, immediately shines."

Joy is a matter of spiritual intelligence for counsellor Paul Edwards. Spiritual intelligence for Edwards, author of *The Spiritual Intelligence Handbook,* is like the intelligence of a genius. "A genius is born, not made. It does not matter how much or how little they know, they are always geniuses. Their genius can never be taken from them. Like genius, spiritual intelligence is a way of thinking. We are all born with it, live with it, and use it. It can never be taken from us. Yet many have not named it and do not have a conscious choice when they use it."

Spiritual intelligence, Edwards asserts, is a scientific fact. "It is true when you are feeling secure, at peace, loved and are happy you will see, hear and act differently than when you are feeling insecure, unhappy and unloved. We all have an inner peace, which we can access by using our conscious spiritual thinking. This is not something you tell others about. You must show them how to do it."

The key is that you cannot access the inner peace through your rational, judgemental, analytic and physical thinking. You have to change to see the unseen by using your conscious, sensing, discerning, awareness of spiritual thinking. The challenge is to get the people out of one way into the other way of thinking before trying to enter the inner peace.

"The missing link for me was to start by actually experiencing the presence of anything," Edwards discloses. "You can close your eyes and feel each other by sensing their presence. You don't really have to close your eyes, but you must change from your rational/physical faculty to your conscious/spiritual faculty. And closing your eyes seems to help."

In order to feel the presence of anything by sensing, start with something familiar, he advises. From there it doesn't take but a moment to sense the presence of thc inner peace.

You will find more such advice in the following pages. Some of it is on how to stay healthy and fit naturally. Taking care of your appearance is increasingly becoming the concern of both sexes. The advice here includes not only on grooming naturally and cheaply but also the possibility of earning a living by making and selling natural herbal cosmetics. We do hope that all these suggestions will contribute to your inner joy.

Luis S.R. Vas and **Anita S.R. Vas**
E-mail: vasluis@hotmail.com

How to Feel Good Physically and Mentally

Everyone has seen how stress can affect the body as well as the mind. We get stuck in traffic and end up with a headache. We experience an acne flare-up just before an important social occasion. Overwork and too much worry can lead to an ulcer or even a heart attack.

As far as scientists are concerned, however a cause-and-effect relationship between stress and disease has been hard to prove...until recently.

Research done during the past 10 years has shown that the mind exerts a real, biochemical influence on the body. Some doctors have suggested that stress plays a contributing role in many diseases, and may influence every physical illness to some extent.

Certainly scientists' findings suggest that our emotions, our personality and how we handle stress can help determine how healthy we are.

Although research in this field is still very new, the major finding so far is that the functioning of the body's immune system can be suppressed by stress. The first proof that this was true came as a result of the Apollo space flights in the late 1960s. Scientists noted that even astronauts in tip-top condition, when faced with re-entry to the earth's atmosphere, showed a depressed immune system function.

Exactly how stress affects the immune system is not fully understood. Research suggests that anxiety and other depressive emotions could immobilise key cells called lymphocytes (disease-fighting white blood cells.)

Experiments done on people experiencing intense stress seem to bear out this theory. Grief, when a spouse dies, is the most stressful event on a chart doctors use to assess how much stress an individual is under.

Researchers have also studied widowers (who do not cope as well as women do after the loss of a spouse) for more clues about the effects of stress.

It has been seen that widowers may get sick more often as they don't take care of themselves, and also show depressed immune system response. In fact, the mortality rate among surviving spouses during the first year after their mate's death is upto six times higher than average.

Divorce seems to produce similar results. Researchers have found big differences in immune functions in a group of divorced or separated women. Certain aspects of the immune system were stronger in the women who were less attached to their ex-husbands or separated for a long time than in those recently separated. And among married women, according to one study, those having marital trouble showed a less vigorous response.

Physical Effects

One of the major ways stress affects the body is through the familiar flight-or-fight response. This is the reaction that gave primitive man that extra burst of power needed to flee a wild animal or face a battle.

What actually happens in the body under stress is an extremely swift series of events. The mind perceives a threat, the brain gets the message and the autonomic nervous system gears up to meet the foe. It doesn't matter that the enemy today is more likely to be a traffic jam than a tiger.

Your heart races, your blood pressure climbs, and blood surges to the muscles in preparation for action. Oxygen and extra nutrients speed to the brain, making you more alert, and secretion of adrenalin, a powerful hormone increases.

When stress is short-term, so are the effects of this sequence of events. But when stress is prolonged-such as during an unhappy marriage or at a miserable job-the effects may linger. In this situation, a series of hormonal reactions takes place, culminating in the release of a hormone called cortisol from the adrenal glands, which suppresses the immune system.

Coping with Stress

Even as we acknowledge the negative effects of stress, we cannot always avoid it, nor should we try to. Would the astronauts have given up the chance to orbit the Earth just because their immune systems were strained on splashdown? Would you avoid moving to a new house or taking a trip just to avoid the possible stress? Restricting stress often means restricting life.

The answer to the dilemma involves minimising the amount of negative stress in your life and learning how to cope with it when it occurs.

Getting fired - or even just changing jobs - is traumatic. But it could be more traumatic for some than for others. Someone harassed by a tyrannical boss, for example, would find changing jobs a positive stress. Not changing jobs would be a negative stress.

It's also how you cope with it that makes the difference. In a study of company executives in high-stress jobs, researchers found that some were sick more often than others. What distinguished the hardy group from the others was the attitude. "They had a clear sense of who they were and about their values," a psychologist said. "The hardy ones made the most of a situation."

Powerful Feelings

The power of repressed emotions to influence health is echoed by a number of doctors who treat patients with classic stress-related illnesses, such as skin and stomach problems.

No matter how painful, feelings themselves cause us less trouble than our efforts to protect ourselves from them. When we don't experience the pain of difficult events—when we don't feel our feelings—we are much more prone to develop physical symptoms.

What kind of physical symptoms a person would develop, appears to depend more on genes than on the type of stress or personality. Everyone has a weak system or organ, usually determined by heredity. The biochemical reactions triggered by stress simply seek out the weakness. For example, if your mother had digestive problems, chances are that you, too, will experience tension in your stomach.

People who are prone to stress may have a variety of symptoms—ulcers, eczema and backache are common ones. Although, these are not the only possibilities, it's helpful to look at what researchers say about them.

The Stomach

While ulcers can be treated successfully with medication, gastroenterologists are now rethinking about the role of stress in many digestive disorders. The reason? Hormones found in the gastrointestinal tract have also been discovered in the brain. This indicates that all diseases of the gastrointestinal tract can be related to stress. These complaints include heart-burn, various forms of colitis, spastic colon and gastritis.

The entire digestive tract is nothing but a series of muscles that become tense. People do not realise they are experiencing tension or, to be precise, muscular contractions, when they want to hit someone but don't, or when they are stuck in traffic at a busy intersection.

The Skin

Shielding organs from outside forces, the skin is linked to the brain by thousand of nerve endings. And it mirrors your emotions. Embarrassment causes you to blush, and fear can make you grow pale.

Even when the cause of skin disease is clearly physical—such as with infection or chemical irritation—most dermatologists agree that stress can trigger outbreaks or make them worse.

Some of you might be aware that your skin disease is aggravated by stress. If conventional treatment hasn't worked, or the condition has returned, you might follow the advice of psychologists who have successfully treated patients with a combination of hypnosis, psychotherapy and visualisation, following the belief that skin disease is often caused by emotional distress.

The Back

Although it has not been fully established, one senior medical researcher has suggested that specific pain syndromes of the neck, shoulders, back and buttocks are caused not by structural abnormalities but by tension. The tension constricts the blood vessels leading to these areas, resulting in muscle spasm and nerve pain.

But then what causes the tension? Above all, back pain is a reflection of temperament. As our lives become more complex, we generate more and more tension.

Treating Stress

A number of treatments based on the mind-over-body principle have been successfully tested against a variety of stress-related conditions.

There is a growing body of evidence-but no definite proof-that they have a positive effect on the immune system. They also produce lower blood pressure, slower heart rate, slower metabolism and relaxation of muscles. And if used daily, they may even protect you from stress by making you less sensitive to it.

These techniques are in no way replacements for traditional medical therapy. Doctors emphasise that they should be used in conjunction with conventional treatment, or when medical therapy has failed.

They are best learned from a qualified instructor, but once mastered, they can be done at home.

The Relaxation Response

This is an inborn mechanism that counteracts the harmful effects of stress. One simple technique involves focussing your mind on a one-syllable word, the sound of your breath, a mantra (for those who have studied transcendental meditation) or even a short prayer for about 10 to 20 minutes.

It is best to do this in a quiet room, in a comfortable position. Most people find sitting in a straight-backed chair works best for them. The key is to let thoughts pass through your mind without dwelling on them.

Progressive Muscle Relaxation

This simple technique consists of producing tension and then relaxing 10 to 20 muscle groups. By doing this, you learn the physical difference between feeling relaxed and feeling tense.

Close your eyes and release as much tension as possible. Then make specific muscles tense (for instance, the abdominal ones) for five seconds while relaxing the rest of your body, and then release tension. Breathe normally, but hold your breath when contracting the muscles of the chest and back, and exhale when you release them. If outside thoughts intrude, try to disregard them and refocus on your breathing.

Hypnosis and Imagery

All hypnosis, in effect, is self-hypnosis, but a professional should first monitor you. For years, skilled hypnotists have put people into trances to treat a number of stress-related illnesses and reduce pain. To learn self-hypnosis, you need a qualified instructor to tailor a programme just for you.

Interested in breaking unwanted habits like smoking and overeating? In developing new skills, say in computer, cricket? In overcoming anxiety of facing an interview, or appearing for exams? In getting over phobias or fears of death, height, water? In tackling personal problems like shyness, loss of a loved one?

Guided imagery and fantasy technique can be used to overcome unwanted habits and improve performance. The guided imagery and fantasy technique relies on the patient being made to use his imagination, preferably under the guidance of a psychotherapist, to change his unwanted habits, improve skills, or overcome fears. This technique is similar to self-hypnosis and is fast gaining popularity as it can be used by the patient himself.

The guided imagery and fantasy technique has to be practised in a state of complete relaxation. The individual must be calm and relaxed for this technique to be effective, or else it would be like day-dreaming.

Let's take the case of a man who wants to give up smoking. The psychiatrist treating the smoker asks him to relax completely. Then some well thought out questions regarding this particular unwanted habit are put to him in rapid succession. The question and answer session follows like this: How would you feel healthwise? Would your food taste better? Will your clothes smell cleaner? And so on.

The individual is then asked to mentally answer these questions as well as visualise himself with a changed and better personality.

Like in this case, the smoker would imagine himself to be a healthier person, with an increased stamina and renewed vigour. The food would definitely taste better and the clothes would smell cleaner then.

The smokers are made to mentally rehearse this situation a number of times. Then gradually they realise the plus points of giving up smoking.

The recent and the most exciting application of guided imagery has been seen in improving an individual's performance in any field. Let's take the case of a sportswoman getting ready to participate in an event. She is asked by the psychiatrist following questions: how she would actually play the game, what are her weak points, where does she need to improve, what exercises and what type of diet does she require, etc. She is then made to even visualise her victory in the game. Another method that the psychiatrist can use is to teach her to visualise a model athlete whom she admired or who possessed the qualities she wants to acquire.

In this case, after answering all these questions, she imagines herself as a better performer. She is then made to rehearse this a number of times—a practice that eventually results in a better performance.

Imagery also helps in healing. Dr. Carl Simmonton has been using imagery on cancer patients in addition to the medical treatment being given to them at the Cancer Counselling Centre at Fortworth, USA. His research shows that patients treated with imagery live longer than patients receiving just medical treatment. The cancer patients are taught to visualise the body defences destroying the cancer cells, building up new cells to replace damaged ones. And the healing and growth of new tissue. All these visualisation techniques do help in reducing pain.

In sport medicine too, guided imagery is used in healing. Here, suppose an athlete has a strained muscle, he is made to visualise healing processes such as the muscle fibres loosening and alighing, the damaged cells being washed away and so on. Finally he is made to visualise that his muscles are firm, elastic, smooth, vibrant and solid.

One important factor that must be kept in mind is that visualisation should be learned and practised under the supervision of a trained professional, so that athletes who practise the self-help technique, do not have any misconceptions about being healed, when they get actually injured.

We use mental imagery on various occasions in our daily lives without realising it. For example, before buying a new outfit, a girl imagines how she will look wearing that particular outfit.

Quite often before delivering a speech, an individual mentally rehearses the points and the language he would use in his speech. This same technique of mental imagery is applied in guided imagery to achieve a specific purpose of either eliminating unwanted habits or in improving performances.

Louie Nassaney, thirty years old, is the only sufferer of the dreaded disease AIDS (Acquired Immune Deficiency Dyndrome) who has been cured by a form of meditation called 'visual imagery.' When Louie discovered he had AIDS, years ago, his health began to deteriorate rapidly. He had constant diarrhoea, fever, weight loss, hallucinations and speech and eyesight impediments. In the beginning of 1984 he was persuaded to stop all medication and start visualization.

He was told to imagine the depleted T-Cells in his bloodstream as little white rabbits, multiplying rapidly. Louie Nassaney regained lost weight, his T-cell count is normal and he has no symptoms of ill health. In fact he looks and feels hundred percent fit.

What is this visual imagery that can work miracle cures when all else has failed? Doctors have long been fascinated by the way the mind produces powerful influence on the body. Sadness causes the lacrimal glands to overflow, causing tears. Danger, whether real or imagined, quickens the heart rate, increases blood sugar content, raises blood pressure and makes the person breathe in a rapid, jerky manner. Anger produces similar symptoms. What doctors found was that emotions were not the only means of causing physiological change. Specific mental pictures can also have a profound effect on the body. Australian psychologist Alan Richardson made the interesting discovery that physical skills can be improved through mental practice.

He asked three groups of young basketball players to participate in an exercise. The first group actually practised shooting free-throws for twenty minutes every day for twenty days. The second group was allowed no practice and the third group was told to 'practise mentally' every day for twenty minutes. They were told to relax and then to visualise themselves taking aim and shooting with great accuracy. All three groups started out with fairly even abilities. The first group which had actually practised shooting, showed a 24 per cent improvement. The second group showed no improvement and the third group that had practised by imagining themselves shooting the basketball, improved by 23 per cent.

Many athletes today practise and use visualisation, thus improving their performance one hundred per cent. Sports psychologist William Morgan claims that elite runners rely on visualization during their long training runs. Some runners say they can train harder by picturing themselves in competition—others prefer to focus on non-competitive images to help them train; the lightness and ease of a gull skimming a blue sky.

Dr. Thaddeus Kistrubala, who uses running as a cure for emotional disorders, asks his patients to visualise themselves as animals—deer or antelopes, or swift running cheetahs—to help them to transfer mental strength to their bodies.

Visualization can help to reduce stress and depression and to invigorate the immune system. Through visualization, smoking can be given up, weight can be lost permanently and self-images improved. The core of all visualization techniques is relaxation. Progressive relaxation improves visualization and makes it more effective. Dr. Carl Simonton, the pioneer in the use of visualization with cancer patients used this technique:

1. Find a quiet room or place without any disturbances. No radios, televisions, or phones.

2. Become aware of your breathing and notice how the diaphragm expands and contracts as you breathe.
3. Make a mental picture of tension in your muscles—see a clenched fist or a tightly contorted facial muscle.
4. Watch the fist open, the face smooth out. Move down the body from head to toes, visualizing tight muscles and seeing them relax and smooth out.
5. Imagine yourself in a beautiful garden, a sunny golden beach, in green, scented woods, or in any place which for you, means peace and happiness. If you don't have such a place invent one.
6. Now picture vividly what you want to happen. If you are an athlete begin your training. If you are a patient, visualise yourself getting well as your body heals itself. One patient with terrible arthritis, pictured an army of small men to smooth and lubricate her stiffened joints. If you have eczema, picture a smooth, clean skin, glowing with fresh blood.

   To be successful, visualisation must be practised for twenty minutes at a time, twice a day. "The subconscious mind doesn't know the difference between the real and the imaginary."

The mind has the power to create pictures that can then become reality. If you are crippled with pain, visualization could be the answer. It all depends on how seriously you take up the project and how sincerely you carry it out.

If visualization is hard for you there is only one solution—practice. Most religions use a great deal of visualization, concentrating on a sacred symbol, yantra, mandala or figure of a God or a teacher to produce a one-dimensional mind. The same principle is used in Creative Visualization. Don't expect instant results. But when you can go into a relaxed state and visualize clearly what is it you want, success can never be far off.

You get into bed, turn out the light and suddenly remember your mother's birthday is the next day and you haven't yet sent her a card.

You are plodding to work through overheated streets and your mind wanders to that hill station vacation you'd love to take and how you might pay for it.

At the dinner table, you suddently hear your son say, "Well, what's your answer?" But you never heard the question because you were having a mental argument with your boss.

Stuck on a long line at the airport, while awaiting your turn you wonder what you'd say or do if your old boyfriend were on the plane.

Daydreams are those thoughts that leap unbidden into your mind. Though they have long been disparaged as signs of hidden hostility, repressed sexuality and neurosis or as simply a waste of time, recent studies of daydreams have shown them to be an extremely useful-perhaps essential-human phenomenon.

Daydreams, these studies show, are not just the idle fluff of an empty mind. They can help you solve current problems, prepare for future events, ward off tension, relieve boredom, dispel fear, dissipate anger and lift depression. They can help to build self-esteem and may even increase the chances for success. Many sport figures spur themselves on to victory by imagining the act of winning.

Even those daydreams that might be described as bizarre fantasies can be useful, perhaps changing bad moods or enhancing self-image. Children who daydream a lot tend to be happier, more cooperative and have longer staying power than those who don't often let their imaginations run away with them, according to studies by Dr. Jerome Singer, a Yale University psychologist and author, with Ellen Switzer, of 'Mind Play.'

Many artists, writers and scientists have their most creative insights through daydreams. Archimedes realised how to use water to measure an object's density while immersing himself in a bathtub. Gazing at the sun setting on the River Seine inspired many of Debussy's Impressionistic compositions.

Yet, Dr. Singer points out, many people are embarrassed by their daydreams or are afraid to let their fantasies unfold. Some repress their daydreams as useless wanderings. Others are so busy they don't take the time for mind-wandering. Still others click on the television to escape through someone else's fantasies, which are not necessarily relevant to their own personal situations.

Daydreams, the studies have shown, are a nearly universal experience that reflect a basic need of the human mind to fill itself with thought.

"Many of the things we do are automatic", says Dr. Eric Klinger, a psychologist at the University of Minnesota. "When we're not using our full thinking capacity, the mind works over other aspects of life. This is an efficient use of our thought spaces."

His studies showed that 30 to 40 per cent of our waking moments are typically spent day dreaming. Most daydreams are just passing thoughts lasting 5 to 14 seconds, such as wondering what to wear to a party. Interspersed are shorter scraps of thought— "I must remember to buy vegetables "and longer reveries lasting perhaps a minute or two."

Research by Dr. Leonard M. Giambra of the National Institute on Aging has shown that, contrary to what you might think, elderly persons immerse in daydreams, mulling over might-have-been or reviving the past. Men aged 75 to 91 daydream as often about the present and future as they do about the past, his studies show. In fact the frequency of daydreams decreases with age, the men over 75 reporting that they daydream only one-fourth as often as males 17 to 23.

But as you might expect, the leading subject on daydreams among young men is sex. For young women, sexual daydreams occur less often. In both sexes, sexual daydreams are most common among those who are most active sexually. Only after about 30 do sexual daydreams of men yield to those of a problem-solving nature.

Females apparently daydream more often than males, with problem-solving daydreams, the most common type of all ages. According to Dr. Klinger's studies, only about one in five daydreams contain weird or distorted images and far fewer represent bizarre flights of fancy.

Dr. Singer points out that there are many ways in which you can make daydreams work to your advantage. The most important use is to play-act your way through problems, rehearsing solutions or reactions to possible future events or situations or carrying out a mental argument until the matter seems settled in your mind. Other possibilities suggested by Dr. Singer include the following:

You can use them simply to fill up time—to amuse yourself, for example, when you have to wait and can do nothing else or when you're driving long distances on a boring road. Since daydreams are associated with a relaxed state, they help to reduce restlessness and tension that could raise your blood pressure or produce other unwanted signs of stress. He cites studies in which persons were enclosed in a booth for a long time and given a "mindless" boring task to do. Those who daydreamed didn't realise how much time had passed.

You can often reverse unpleasant moods and counter feelings of depression with "positive" fantasies, especially those that enhance self-esteem, such as day-dreams in which you imagine yourself winning an Oscar or the U.S. Open or being named President of the company. Daydreams about happy events, joyful feelings or peaceful scenes can relax the muscles of your head and perhaps even ward off tension and headaches.

Bizarre fantasies can help to diminish anger. Let's say you're angry with the boss for not giving you a raise and you're about to confront the matter head-on. Since anger may not be the best emotion for such a confrontation, you could dissipate it by imagining the boss surprising you with a present and giving you a promotion and a raise or by picturing the boss standing up to shake your hand.

Athletes and musicians who engage in fantasy practice—as well as physically practising their skills, tend to do better in carrying them out. Daydreams about other activities may also help you perform them better.

If you have phobias, you can use daydreams to diminish your fear. For example, if you are afraid of flying, you can imagine yourself on the plane talking to a fascinating seatmate or reading a racy novel and having a wonderful time. If you're frightened about taking a test, you can daydream about something pleasant and peaceful and calm yourself down. By the same token, however, if you allow your daydreams to picture the worst (a plane crash or failing in the test) you could greatly enhance your fears.

Daydreams can sometimes be a clue to an important problem that is not being resolved or failing in a need not being met. For example, one Madison Avenue advertising executive found himself constantly daydreaming about sailing. He finally decided to invest in a charter yacht and is now happy as a lark running a business in the Caribbean. If you find that daydreams constantly intrude at inappropriate times, it could be a sign that something is wrong in your life and professional guidance may be needed.

Why do some people get sick? Why does illness strike at one time and not at another?

According to authors June Bingham and Dr. Norman Tamarkin, in their book **The Pursuit of Health,** the answers to these intriguing questions can be linked to what they call the Intimate Connector (IC).

This force, which includes 'spirit' and 'soul', 'character' and 'personality', is constantly organising and reorganising the four dimensions of each person's health:

- body
- mind
- relationships with other people;
- relationships with environments, social and ethical as well as physical

Each dimension continually interacts with the other three, the authors say. If we have a problem with our boss (other people), it may show up as a pain in the neck (body) or as a chronic anxiety (mind). On the other hand, the problem may be resolved because we talk about it with a friend (other people) or please our boss by finding a faster route to work (environment).

Good health, according to the authors, is a wholesome cycle. You wake up feeling fine, you work or play, you relax alone or with a loved one in the evening, you sleep well and wake up feeling fine, perhaps even better.

Poor health is likely to be one of two things: either the merely temporary interruption of a characteristically wholesome cycle or the beginning of a vicious cycle. Because human health operates as an integrated system, a vicious cycle can be interrupted either in the dimension where the symptom first arose or in any of the others. Treatment in some dimension other than the original one may speed recovery.

For the lucky individual with good genes and a well functioning IC, to remain fit takes little effort: It's doing what comes naturally. For someone less fortunate, or at a less favourable stage, a minor ailment in one dimension may set in motion troublesome reactions in other dimensions.

The authors, of course, acknowledge the old adage that prevention is far better than cure, so they have recommended a series of rules to maintain generally good health, plus a set of warning signs that either warn you of the approach of something drastic, or reassure you that the symptoms you believe you have are not as you might think.

Depression Signals

If, for no evident reason, more than six of the following symptoms develop, the person should check with a doctor in regard to depression:

1. Feeling of sadness, hopelessness ("I will never improve.")
2. Loss of pleasure capacity, 'the ability to enjoy.'
3. Loss of usual interest in sex.
4. Loss of appetite (or overeating).
5. Insomnia (or sleeping too much)
6. Anxious or restless behaviour (orapathy).
7. Difficulty in concentration, memory, decision-making.
8. Becoming unduly upset by small things.
9. Feelings of worthlessness ("I'm no good.")
10. Withdrawal from friends and relatives.

Signals that may Indicate Cancer

1. Uncharacteristic constipation (or perhaps diarrhoea) gas pains, severe indigestion, loss of appetite, rectal bleeding.
2. In the mouth, painless sore or a raised, irregular warty area; a lump or thickening of the cheek, gum, or tongue.

3. Difficulty in swallowing, persistent hoarseness; a lump in the throat.
4. On the skin, a sore that does not heal, a dry, scaly patch, a pimple that persists, an inflamed area with a crusting centre, or a pale, waxy, pearly nodule.
5. In the lungs a cough that persists.
6. For men: any continuing urinary difficulty, lower back, pelvic or upper thigh pain, blood in urine (also a danger signal for women).
7. For women: Unusual bleeding or discharge from the vagina; any lump or thickening or unusual puckering of the skin of the breast.

Commonsense Rules of Diet

1. Avoid excess salts and sugar.
2. Keep low the consumption of red meat, primarily beef and lamb and substitute fish and poultry, legumes and grains, nuts and seeds.
3. Substitute low-fat milk for whole milk, low-fat cheese for high-fat cheese.
4. Substitute polyunsaturated margarine and vegetable oils for butter, lard and bacon fat.
5. Eat plenty of fruits, and green leafy, as well as yellow vegetables, raw and cooked.

General Health

1. Get seven or eight hours' sleep at night.
2. Eat breakfast-especially highfibre foods and fruits.
3. Keep weight normal in relation to height.
4. Avoid smoking.
5. Exercise regularly.
6. Drink only in moderation (a glass or two of wine or beer per day and spirits only occasionally).
7. Burn the candle at only one end (*i.e.,* if you work too hard, then don't play too hard, or if you play too hard, then don't work too hard; alternate periods of overexertion with periods of rest, and periods of laziness with periods of self-galvanishing).

Facts for the Emergency Room

Any day-or night-you could become one of the thousands of people who are rushed to hospitals every month for emergency treatment. And a trip to the hospital is usually the sort of thing that happens just when you least expect it.

So what can you do about it? Be prepared, wherever you are, with the answers hospital personnel need to speed your case.

In short, carry with you at all times certain basic information that can be of vital importance when every minute counts. Our research indicates you should have:

1. Your name, address, phone number, physical description, and identifying marks (perhaps even a passport-type photo), and information on your doctor and others to notify in the event of an emergency.
2. Your occupation and your employer's name, address, and phone number, if you have it; the name and address of a responsible party, and information on any hospital insurance you have.
3. A quick checklist giving your blood type, allergies and/or drug sensitivities; immunisations (including the date of your last tetanus booster); notice if you have a history of such problems as heart trouble, diabetes or epilepsy and a notation of any organs removed or any implants.
4. Brief details on your current medication (including dosage and precise identification of drugs); comments on significant medical problems; your surgical history (including dates and doctors).

   This material should be clearly identified, organised as precisely as possible and should be readily available.

   The trouble you take in preparing it will be more than compensated by the knowledge that it might well be of key importance in speeding your admission, diagnosis, treatment, and recovery.

Dieting Tips for Quitters

Heart authorities, aware of the fact that many smokers, especially women, fear they will gain weight if they give up smoking, have issued several tips about weight control. Among them are:

- Choose foods that keep your hands busy, such as unshelled nuts.
- Chew sugarless gum.
- Use artificially sweetened mints.
- For snacks, keep a supply of cut raw vegetables and unbuttered popcorn.
- Keep high calorie foods out of the house if possible, and certainly out of sight.
- Have someone else put away the leftovers.
- Slow down your eating by cutting food into smaller pieces, putting the fork down between bites, sipping water.
- Temporarily avoid alcohol, which adds calories and diminishes will-power.
- Exercise.

It wasn't very long ago that walking was considered the world's most popular (and only) mass transit system, but not anymore.

In today's world of subways and space shuttles, walking has quite suddenly re-merged as a mass health-regeneration system.

A regular walking programme can help you lose weight, give you more energy and tone your flabby muscles. It can help prevent heart disease, relieve the pain of angina, alleviate mental depression and ease some of the pain of arthritis as well as reverse some of the physical aspects of aging.

It's hard to believe that something as simple as walking can really produce all these benefits, but scientists are beginning to find that the world's oldest form of aerobic exercise may really be the best. Take its effect on weight loss, for example.

"Regular exercise can be the single most useful thing a moderately obese person can do to lose weight," says Joel Grinker, Ph.D., professor of nutrition in the School of Public Health and Pediatrics at the University of Michigan. "I tell almost everyone that walking is the best exercise they can get, because it doesn't stress the body the way running does. Swimming is good, too", she adds, "but you need a pool for that."

Walking Vs Dieting

Some would argue, why go for all the trouble? Why not just go on a diet to lose weight?

"For one thing, with exercise you don't suffer the decrease in metabolic rate that accompanies severe calorie restriction," says Dr. Grinker, who heads the programme in human nutrition at the university. She explains that stringent dieting lowers the body's metabolism, which means that proportionately fewer calories are burned. But exercise helps to increase the metabolic rate, meaning that more calories are being burned up over a longer period of time.

There have been many studies showing that exercise is more effective than dieting for losing weight. In one, Grant Gwinup, M.D., assembled a group of obese people in California who had all failed to lose weight by dieting. Dr. Gwinup asked them to continue their normal eating habits but to walk at least 30 minutes or more per day for a year. At the end of a year, all of the subjects had lost weight, averaging 10 kgs each.

One of the big advantages to walking is the kind of weight you lose. If you're walking off the bulges, you'll be getting rid of fat, whereas dieting also causes loss of lean body tissue, or muscle.

There is little doubt among health care professionals today that when reasonable eating habits are combined with exercise, such as walking, weight loss is more rapid than when either method is used alone. And with walking you won't get the feelings of weakness and nervousness that go along with dieting.

Heart Benefits

While you're walking off unwanted pounds, you'll be doing your heart a favour, too. For many sedentary and older people, brisk walking at a pace of four to five miles per hour can provide a workout for the heart and lungs comparable to that of jogging, according to Robert Kertzer, Ph.D. Dr. Kertzer incorporates walking into a special cardiac rehabilitation programme at the University of New Hampshire.

"If the activity is rhythmic, involves a large percentage of the body's musculature and is continuous, it's good for cardiovascular fitness," says Dr. Kertzer, who is an associate professor of Physical Education.

Joseph Tenenbaum, M.D., a cardiologist and assistant professor of clinical medicine at Columbia University's Medical School in Manhattan, concurs—

"The key to therapeutic walking is consistent rhythm in exercise, with major muscle groups kept in action for 30 minutes at least four times a week," he says. "I recommended walking to a lot of my patients."

Many of Dr. Tenenbaum's patients are in the healing phase following a heart attack, and he feels that walking is the ideal exercise for them or anyone who is convalescing to rebuild strength. In fact, Dr. Tenenbaum's patients may be preventing future heart attacks with their walking programmes.

Sixty-four patients who had been recommended for coronary-bypass surgery by their personal physicians chose it instead of trying lifestyle modifications. They entered the Pritikin Longevity Centre in California for a 26-day session. There, in addition to following the Pritikin high-complex-carbohydrate, high-fibre, low-fat diet, they participated in a walking programme of two brisk walks per day, each lasting 30 to 45 minutes.

At the end of the 26 days, all of the subjects had lost weight, their blood pressures had decreased, their surum-cholesterol and triglyceride levels were significantly reduced, and in some cases, angina was relieved. Five years later, those who continued to follow the programme's guidelines at home were still benefiting from it. In fact their mortality rate was actually approaching that of the general population.

Good eating habits unquestionably played a role in these patients' progress, but exercise can help prevent heart problems without any dietary modifications. The American Heart Association, for example, suggests that regular exercise, such as walking, may protect against heart disease.

Even extremely moderate walking, at a pace too slow to provide the cardiovascular benefits of a brisk walk, can raise HDL-C levels. Since people with low levels of HDL-C (high-density-lipo-protein-cholesterol) are considered to be especially vulnerable to heart attacks, they'd be well advised to get out for daily strolls. In a recent University of Pittsburgh School of Medicine study, 30 sedentary men exercised at three different levels rose just as sharply during low-intensity exercises as they did in high-intensty sessions. But if slow walking is better than no walking, fast walking is the best.

"Just being on your feet and moving from point A to point B is not equivalent to an exercise programme," warns Dr. Tenenbaum. "Window shopping, for example, or just moving around at work can't substitute for a brisk daily walk."

The reason most health-care professionals recommend setting a vigorous pace during your walking workout is because there seems to be a threshold in the intensity of exercise that must be reached to provide for improvements in the heart and circulation. Fast walking, like any aerobic exercise, will enable your heart to beat fewer times, since it is pumping more blood with each beat.

As if strengthening your heart and keeping you trim weren't enough, walking can promote metabolic changes that may help prevent or manage adult-onset diabetes mellitus by inducing an insulin-like effect on cellular-glucose uptake. Furthermore, walking can help to heal bone loss, thereby preventing osteoporosis. And since exercise has been shown to slow degenerative joint changes, walking can prevent or relieve some symptoms of rhematoid arthritis.

In fact, as far as joints are concerned, walking is frequently the best exercise.

"If a person has a damaged joint or ligament, or the kind of back problem that might be aggravated by jolting, then running may be bad for that person," says Robert Leach, M.D., professor and Chairman of Orthopaedic surgery at Boston University Medical School.

"Even walking produces some impact when the heel strikes the ground, but there is no question that jogging produces more impact force. That won't harm a normal joint, but a disabled joint is better off walking," advises Dr. Leach, who has had plenty of opportunity to study the effect of impact on joints in his capacity as consultant to the Boston Celtics, head physician to the summer-Olympic teams in Los Angeles in 1984 and orthopaedic surgeon to Olympic gold-medal marathoner Joan Benoit.

"Walking is a very efficient exercise," Dr. Leach asserts, "especially in terms of toning muscles and giving people a good feeling."

Help for the Depressed

Psychiatrists, particularly, are beginning to recognize the value of the "good feeling" Dr. Leach refers to. Walking, like jogging, appears to promote increased endorphin production (endorphins are neurohormones that may produce a sense of well-being).

"I recommended brisk walking-rapid enough to condition the heart-for all my patients who are depressed or suffering from low self-esteem," says Ralph Wharton, M.D., a psychiatrist in New York who specializes in the treatment of depression. "Even 20 or 30 minutes a day seems to make a difference. For one thing, going for a walk prevents excessive preoccupation and rumination, and it distracts you from your own inner concerns."

If one of the things that depresses you is the thought of aging, you've got all the more reason to start walking. In a programme involving a group of Canadian men and women in their mid-60s who were given endurance training that emphasized vigorous walking, several interesting results were achieved. Body fat was decreased, knee extension capabilities were increased, body potassium levels were increased and the normal age-related loss of bone calcium was apparently halted. In other words, the best way to reach the fountain of youth is to walk there at a brisk pace.

In addition to all the good things walking can do for you physically and emotionally, it can also improve your social life by introducing you to new people and new experiences. Many organisations sponsor walks ranging from leisurely to strenuous that attract people with many varied interests. Even urban areas sometimes offer excellent walks for the resident or visitor to participate in.

"After all, if you're going to put up with the problems of a city, you deserve some of its pleasures", says Howard Goldberg, whose organization 'Adventure on a Shoestring' has been conducting people on fascinating walks around Manhattan for 22 years. To find out if a city you're planning to visit offers walking tours, Goldberg suggests contacting the local visitor's bureau. In India there could be a great future for such tours.

To set up your own daily walking programme, consult your doctor first if you have pain or haven't had a check up for some time. Once you've got the go ahead, get yourself a pair of comfortable, flexible walking (or running) shoes, preferably with cushioned soles. Start off slowly if you're in poor physical condition, building up to as fast a pace as you can handle. Walk at least 30 minutes a day, three or four days a week. In extremely hot or cold weather, walk in a shopping centre in the halls of your apartment building or around a track in a gym. Go walking by yourself or with a friend, or get a group together. As well as being good exercise, walking can be just plain fun—and that's the best medicine of all!

"The faster you walk, the better you can feel," says Howard Jacobson, executive director of the Walkers Club of America.

Jacobson's aim is to get us all health walking, an activity that he says is best accomplished by pumping your arms vigorously while you walk. Health walking is a non-competitive form of race walking, a venerable sport that has been an Olympic event since 1908.

"By moving your arms like a sprinter, you can move faster, which will raise your heart rate higher than normal walking," Jacobson says. "And you'll be using more muscles and burning more calories than joggers, with less risk of injury."

How does the novice start healthy walking? Jacobson recommends walking rapidly in a normal way but with your arms pumping like a sprinter's. Avoid swaying from side to side, he says, because that slows you down.

Jacobson, a coach to Olympians and author of **Racewalk to Fitness** emphasizes that health walking can be done by almost everyone, at any age. Young children in Sweden race walk in school programmes. In the United States, 93-year old Gwen Clark health walks six miles every day in New York's Central Park. So, if you want to take up health walking yourself, you won't be alone.

Natural Health and Fitness

A wide range of techniques, both Eastern and Western, are designed to make the most of physical effort and body awareness.

Broader in scope than aerobics and gym workouts, they include not only exercises for general fitness but also techniques for freeing specific muscle spasms, correcting poor posture and using the flow of life-force through the body.

It also includes cathartic techniques to release emotional trauma trapped in the musculature of the body.

Like any machine, the body requires lubrication, fuel and rest. An engine is not expected to run continuously without maintenance. So often we allow our health to run down until there is a crisis situation where surgery or potent suppressive drugs are required.

Exercise patterns, too, need to be balanced. You can follow an active, Western yang-type programme (tennis, jogging, swimming, cycling, squash, gym or working out with weights), and harmonise this with yin-type activities such as yoga, breathing and meditation as well.

These 'static' movements may appear non-productive, but they have deep-reaching effects on the muscles, glands and emotions as well as the autonomic nervous system as a whole.

A principle we often forget is that to master an exercise, very, very slowly in order to involve the mind and breath as well as movement, gives one the control to do it at speed. Whereas to use a repetitive movement at speed, perhaps to the rhythm or music, tones the skeletal and vascular systems wonderfully but does little for the integration of mind, body and spirit. A fusion of the knowledge of the two great cultures is what we need to bear in mind.

Here we discuss how to do the gentler of the yang-type exercises, and we look at the more complex yin activities.

Stretching

Try this at frequent intervals during the day as a general energy booster and release to tension. You can also circle the shoulders backwards, and forwards and roll the head slowly. The aim is to make the muscles elastic.

Stretch the neck up from the shoulders, as if you were being pulled from the crown of the head. Using the top of the neck as a pivot (and not the collar bone), nod the head chin-to-neck in a forward direction and then sideways to each shoulder. Be very careful not to raise the shoulder or bend the head from side to side. It remains on the same plane.

The aim is to achieve an effortless 180 degree-turn and the ability at any age to line up the nose with the shoulder.

The Stomach Lift

The 'ultimate' exercise we should choose, if we had to, is the stomach lift or **uddiyana bandha** of the yogis. It looks after the two main body functions of digestion and elimination, as well as keeping a trim waistline by exercising the vertical rectus abdominis muscles and the oblique abdominals.

This must be done on an empty stomach. So the morning before breakfast is a good time to do it. You can have the added benefit of warm water on your neck and back.

Stand with your feet about 45 cm apart. Bend slightly forward, round the back, bend the knees and place your palms, on your thighs with the fingers pointing inwards. Exhale completely, emptying the lungs, then pull the abdomen upward and backward making the midsection as concave as possible. Remember to leave the lungs empty while you do this and resist the instinct to breathe in when you draw the tummy in. Hold the stomach in with the breath out as long as comfortable (at least to a count of five, to begin with)—then slowly release and breathe in.

At first, to isolate the muscles you are using, place one fist under the rib cage to encourage the tummy tuck right up and under. Repeat at least 10 times.

The Rib Roll

Add this to your morning tune-up: leaning forward, spread the fingers on both hands and tuck them under the length of one side of the rib-cage. On an exhalation press the fingers up under the ribs. Hold for three seconds. Move to the other side and repeat. Finally, placing both forefingers underneath, exhale, lean, forward and press inwards for three seconds. Some areas may be tender from time to time but the pressure helps to clear energy blockages. This daily check also keeps you in touch with the amount of flesh you are carrying over your ribs and midriff!

Massage is the simplest, most natural form of healing.

In ancient times, as well as in the modern era, a mother would rub a baby's tummy if it had colic, a friend would knead and squizze your stiff shoulder muscles, and if you fell and bruised your knee, you would hold the sore spot.

Many people have a massage regularly to maintain health and well-being. There are almost as many massage styles as there are masseurs.

Massage has existed in one form or another for thousands of years. Members of the medical profession now acknowledge the healing and rejuvenating powers of the human touch. According to them, massage increases the circulation of blood, loosens up muscles for easier exercise-and it's very soothing.

When you hurt yourself, your natural response is to take the injured part of your body in your hand. A massage therapist's work is based on this principle. Touching is an important part of aiding the system in its own repair and maintenance. The restorative touch of the licensed massage therapist is guided by hours of study in the sciences of anatomy, physiology and pathology.

The massaging manipulation breaks down deposits of the chemical by-products of exercise, such as lactic acid, which, when trapped in muscles, leave them sore and stiff. It also reduces any inflammation from muscle injury. Some authorities even believe that massage induces the central nervous system to release endorphins, the body's natural tranquilizers. A once-a-week massage can unwrap layers of tension built up over years.

Should you be alarmed if an occasional move on the part of your massage therapist makes you wince? Sometimes you will feel pain because you are resisting the touch. Or you may start out feeling a little pain, just like when you start exercising. But any discomfort you feel shouldn't be unbearable.

Massage Methods

There are many types of massage available. First, there is the highly specialized probing of the physical therapist, who works in conjunction with doctors to restore injured muscles, tendons and ligaments. Then there is the traditional Swedish massage, which uses long, deep strokes directed towards the heart to improve muscle tone and stimulate circulation. Shiatsu involves the application of pressure with a finger, the palm or the point of an elbow on the acupuncture points of the body to free the energy blockages that translate into muscle tension.

To Give Massage

Once aware of its pleasures, you may be inspired to give a massage to a friend. It's fine to rub the back, arms and feet as long as you do it gently. To give a massage, you need vegetable oil (not baby oil) or a light cleansing cream (which has the advantage of not staining sheets) and a firm surface. Never exert direct pressure on the spine, and never give a massage to someone with varicose veins or arthritis. Pregnant women and people with heart disease or high blood pressure should consult their physicians before having a massage.

How to Rub Yourself the Right Way

The following three simple techniques will help ease pain and leave you feeling refreshed.

For Headaches

With the thumb and index finger of one hand, squeeze the point where the index finger and thumb of the other hand meet in a V shape. Hold for 15 secs. Switch hands and repeat the process.

For Eyestrain

One : place your finger-tips on your forehead, just under the hairline. Place both thumbs on the bridge of your nose. Slowly move your thumbs toward your temples, along the bone under the eyebrows, exerting gentle pressure as you go along. Two : put your thumbs under your jaw. With your index fingers, gently press down all along the ridge of bone under your eyes. This exercise can be done while sitting at your desk, but works best when you're lying down.

For a Pain in the Neck

Place your thumbs on the bones at the base of your skull, applying pressure in a circular motion. Continue in the same way around the jaw. Last, gently massage the outsides of the temples.

It is not concerned with moving particular muscles or joints per se, but with using motion in muscles and joints to produce particular sensor feelings—positive, pleasurable feelings which enter the central nervous system and begin to trigger tissue changes by means of the many sensory-motor feedback loops between the mind and the muscles.

Rather than working for local tissue changes which eventually accumulate to influence physical and mental function, the Trager approach seeks to influence specifically the feeling states in the sensory and the unconscious elements of the mind which most directly control tissue response, metabolism, posture and behavioural patterns.

Since birth, our day-to-day lifestyle has given us all many good and bad experiences. These have shaped us physically and psychologically.

Since it is not possible to avoid all traumas, and since none may be erased once they have occurred, therapy should be directed towards bringing appropriate positive feeling experiences to the patient.

These help to influence the mind and body directly so that the physical patterns can be alleviated. We are all familiar with the degenerative effects that negative feelings and attitudes can have upon the body but it is possible to turn this potent force of feelings to a constructive purpose.

Dr. Trager contends that he is not a healer or a manipulator of esoteric energies, and his successes have nothing miraculous about them.

The kinds of reflex responses, tissue changes, and behavioral changes he is able to elicit are possible because of the intimate neurological associations between sensory stimulations, emotional feelings, attitudes and concepts, and the body's motor responses to them.

Yoga can be useful in reducing stress.

It provides a safe space for subjecting ourselves to a form of 'therapeutic' stress. This 'stretches' us and allows us to let go and experience a sense of freedom.

While doing yoga we can notice our 'normal' reactions to stress. We also learn new ways of dealing with it—correct breathing, strengthening of legs and lower back rather than holding on with the chest and shoulders.

Morning is a good time to practise yoga because the body is rested and refreshed.

In the morning before breakfast the body has more energy but is generally less supple. Before the evening meal you may relieve the tension of the day.

You should practise yoga on an empty stomach.

To look your best you must first be healthy.

Simple 'touch' techniques can help eliminate minor ailments and form the basis of preventive health care.

The 'touch' therapies first began to gain widespread respect and acceptance during the Seventies with healing therapies.

Acupressure and the general reflex therapies are among the most effective means of using nature's healing methods to keep the body functioning at its best.

They do not require pills, drugs, tranquilisers or surgery, and can be administered with safety anywhere or any time by anyone on yourself or on others.

By daily checking for tender areas on the body and gently easing away the blockage of energy with has caused them, future problems can be prevented.

To understand how this is possible, it is useful to study the pathways of the body's energy lines. These are allied to the nervous system, but separate and distinct from it.

When the reflex centres are massaged, a surge of energy is generated along the neutral and meridian lines to the related part of the body and eventually to the associated organ. This primary flow of energy strengthens the body's own healing and defence mechanisms instantly.

Rebirthing

Rebirthing is a breathing process aimed at expanding awareness of, and union with one's inner self, a process that results in healing.

The name 'Rebirthing' conjures up images of being 'reborn' or living through the birth trauma.

In this there are three important elements: breathing, relaxing and awareness.

When we breathe normally, there is an inhalation-pause-exhalation-pause-inhalation.

With the Rebirthing it is inhale-exhale-inhale-exhale. This type of breathing is called connected breathing.

The breathing develops into a circular rhythm, with the active emphasis on the inhalation, and the feeling of relaxation on the exhalation.

By relaxing, a person lets go of the conditioning and reconnects with the innate perfect self.

It is when the reconnection with self takes place that a profound healing occurs.

As deeper and deeper states of relaxation are achieved, thoughts and memories from the unconscious mind become accessible.

Another concept fundamental to rebirthing is accepting personal responsibility.

Until a person accepts responsibility for her situation, it is not possible for her to be able to change it.

A typical breath-session usually lasts for one to two hours.

During the session, the person lies on a bed, gets into a state of relaxation and then beings to breathe rhythmically.

As the breathing proceeds, the energy level gradually rises, and the person may experience symptoms of hypertension, dizziness tingling, cramping, drowsiness or 'going cold.'

Then there is a release of discomfort resulting in a deep state of relaxation and euphoria.

Good Posture conjures up old-fashioned connotations such as a picture of someone standing on her toes, head held high, doing a balancing act with a stack of books on her head! In reality, very few of us have the patience to attempt such a laborious task.

Nevertheless, how you carry yourself does matter, for perfect posture can prevent untold health problems.

The most common faults are slouching round shoulders, sway backs (especially common in women who frequently wear high heels) and holding the head wrongly. Many of us have less obvious defects too. The habit of carrying a shoulder bag, for example, can make one shoulder higher than the other, which puts the body out of line.

And, quite apart from the fact that postural faults like these are unattractive, they're also a health hazard.

Donald Norfolk, a London osteopath and author of **Farewell to Fatigue** sees such defects as "major functional catastrophes leading to tension, tiredness and premature joint decay."

Bad posture is a drain on energy and can cause all sorts of problems, from indigestion to anxiety-related illnesses, and leads to aches and pains-back pain in particular—caused by putting stress on the wrong muscles.

Standing and sitting badly cramps the internal organs and prevents them from working at full, efficient capacity. Slouching cramps the rib cage, for example, which means that the sloucher will have shallow breathing.

A fact to bear in mind: many of us will have shortened by five centimetres by the time we are 50—thanks mainly to a bad posture.

One of the most vulnerable parts of the body is the region where the back of the neck joins the back itself. It is here that faulty posture and distortion often start; and it is here that about 85 per cent of us will suffer from arthritis in our 50s.

When the head is held correctly above the shoulders, the neck gives no trouble. But if we adjust our heads forward, and modern life means we're straining forward a great deal of the time—driving, reading, working at a desk and so on—then the neck muscles have to contract to support the weight. Get the head right-that is, back and evenly balanced on the neck.

Stand with your back to a wall and your feet (take your shoes off) about 10 cm from the skirting board. Your head, shoulder blades and bottom should all make easy contact with the wall, leaving a gap in small of the back just big enough to take the flat of your hand. The spine is meant to curve slightly, but if it curves too much, your head will be thrust forward from the wall.

Learning the right way to stand—and sit and move—is one of the best beauty treatments a woman can give herself. Good posture helps the body to function well, encourages good breathing and guards against premature degeneration. It makes you look slimmer, releases more energy, and gives you a feeling of freedom, because the muscles are working in harmony, and it makes you look more confident.

Stand sideways in front of a mirror with feet slightly apart. Sway slightly forward, putting your weight on your toes, then backwards so that your weight is on your heels. Now "centre" your weight so that it runs through middle of your feet at a point just in front of your ankles.

Next, practise the "pelvic tilt." Bend knees and place one hand on your tummy, the other on the small of your back. Slowly tilt your pelvis forward so that your pubic bone lifts up at the front. Then tilt it backwards so that your bottom sticks out. After tilting forward and back a few times, "centre" your pelvis between the two extremes and straighten your knees, but do not lock them.

Now lift your breastbone—feel your ribs lift up and away from your hips as you do so, helping to get rid of that midriff slump and pot belly. Lift your shoulders slightly and circle them backwards, keeping them low and relaxed.

Your arms should hang loosely, hands just to the front of your thighs.

Your chin should be roughly at right angles to your back. "Think" your neck long, particularly the back of your neck, by imagining the crown of your head is attached to a thread gently pulling you upwards. The feeling should be one of lengthening and stretching, of space between the ribs in the waist and in the hips.

Weak muscles are often responsible for poor posture—and vice versa. Concentrate on toning and strengthening the back and stomach-strong stomach muscles act like a corset and take the strain from back muscles.

A simple exercise that can be done anytime, anywhere, is to pull in your stomach hard, hold for a few seconds, then, release. Sit ups—lying on the floor with knees bent, arms crossed over the chest or behind your head-are well-established tummy-toners.

Any stretching exercises-even a deliberate over-head stretch as if you were trying to reach an apple in a tree—help counteract a tendency to slump. And exercise in general helps release tension build-up in the muscles. Inactivity encourages the body to "set" into its distortions, leading to stiff joints and inflexibility. Swimming is the safest and best exercise for the back.

Look critically at the furniture you use regularly—at home, at work or in your car—and see if any changes need to be made.

Chairs should be firm rather than too soft, give support to the small of your back, and with the seat at a height that allows you to work comfortably with your feet firmly on the floor. Always sit well supported.

When using a table or desk, pivot forward from the hips instead of hunching over with a rounded spine. A sloping work surface, such as that used by draughtsmen and commercial artists, is often more comfortable—improvise with a board proposed on books or blocks.

Generally, 7 cm below is the most comfortable height for a worktop. If it's too low, causing you to stoop, you may be able to adjust the height with blocks of wood. If it's a bit too high, it could be worth having a special board to stand on for lengthy chores.

You should experiment to find what suits you best.

Mattresses should be neither too soft nor too hard—a good one will support you firmly while moulding itself gently to the curve of your spine, making for a good, healthy sleep.

Fatigue can be an early clue that your emotions are out of kilter. It can also be a signal of a physical illness.

We've assembled a list of nine of the most common causes of fatigue. If you feel run-down here's the low-down.

Not Enough Sleep

It seems so obvious, but if you haven't slept well the night before, you're very likely going to feel tired the day after.

Scientists believe sleep disturbance is a common response to changes in our lives, from trouble at the office to serious illness. For most of us, normal sleep patterns return after the daytime problem that is the source of worry goes away or gets better.

If occasional sleeplessness troubles you, follow these simple suggestions from Ms. Patricia Prinz, Ph.D., associate professor of psychiatry and behavioral sciences at the University of Washington School of Medicine, USA.

- Try not to drink coffee or other caffeine drinks after 6 or 7 p.m.
- Go to bed at the same time every night.
- Get regular, moderate exercise.
- Better skip alcohol after dinner. It interferes with sound sleep.

Poor Nutrition

Diet or not, you have to eat if you don't want to wind up nose down on the pavement. Simply put, crash or fad diets can leave you feeling fatigued.

Because they offer so little in the way of balanced nutrition, crash diets can turn your muscle mass into mush. The destruction becomes so pronounced, after a short time, that the muscle tissue can no longer efficiently process calcium, according to recent studies done at the University of Toronto. If you're on that kind of a diet, your body will not be able to function properly. It will slow down and conserve energy by making you slow down.

To get a good start on a diet that will leave you feeling fresh and exhilarated, bear in mind these basic rules:

- Eat a variety of foods. Avoid diet plans that force you to live on one specific kind of food, like grapefruit. We need a wide variety of nutrients from all kinds of food. No one food supplies you with all the nutrients your body needs to maintain health.
- Women in general, shouldn't eat fewer than 1,800 calories a day; men, not less than 1,500 calories. According to diet and nutrition experts at Stanford University, you can't get all the nutrients you need if you get less than those amounts. Diets in the super-low 800 calorie range may pose a particular threat to health which can result in a breakdown in heart muscle.
- If you cut 250 calories a day from your diet, you should lose about a half pound a week.
- Don't eat big meals late at night. You probably won't be able to burn off the calories as quickly by bedtime as you would earlier in the day.
- Don't skip meals. If you do, you'll only be hungrier later. When you sit down to eat, you probably will eat more than you should.

Lack of Exercise

If your body isn't exercised regularly, it probably doesn't use oxygen very efficiently. Your muscles need that oxygen, or they don't work as long or as hard as they can. The result of all this sitting around: when you need muscle power, you don't get it, and you tire quickly.

What's more, even as your muscles sag, so, too, does your self-image. Your emotional state can become a mirror image of your physical condition, adding to your fatigue.

That's why exercise benefits you in two ways. First, it improves your physical condition, enabling your body to deliver oxygen more efficiently to your muscles, increasing your endurance. Second, exercise stimulates an overall feeling of well-being.

Studies show that as you exercise, your body is able to handle better the everyday emotional and physical stresses of life, says Ralph Wharton, M.D., clinical professor of psychiatry at Columbia University. "The question is, what does exercise do in a neurochemical sense? We don't know exactly," he says. "But we do know that, whatever exercise does for the brain, it also seems to do for the ego. When people exercise, they see themselves running or swimming well. They feel a certain mastery of the environment."

Drug Reactions

You get plenty of sleep, you jog around the park, but you feel exhausted, like you just can't get started. May be your fatigue is coming from outside your body.

A number of drugs—including antihistamines, pain relievers, diuretics, antihypertensive, antibiotics, oral contraceptives and anticonvulsants—can sometimes cause fatigue as a side-effect.

If you are taking a drug and you think it makes you feel drowsy, the first thing to do is to call the pharmacist who sold you the product, says William N Tindall, Ph.D., Director of Professional Affairs for the National Association of Retail Druggists.

Your doctor will have your complete drug history and will be able to tell whether the drug you are taking is causing your drowsiness, or whether two drugs in combination are having that effect.

What he might do, says Dr. Tindall, is substitute another drug. "With all the drugs on the market, they can usually find something that isn't as hard on the patient."

Whatever you do, don't stop taking a prescription drug without consulting your physician first.

Stress

It takes a lot of energy to deal with the pressures of everyday life. After expending all that energy, you may be left with a gnawing, overwhelming sense of fatigue.

Not all the stresses of life leave us feeling emotionally drained. "It takes a certain kind of stress, in which you have no choices, no options, no alternatives," says Harvey L Alpern, M.D., a board certified cardiologist in Los Angeles.

"The classic example is the woman who finds herself in a dead-end job. She has a tough boss that she can't talk back to. She has to do the same, repetitive things, day after day. She has no sense of control. She may have a family who needs her, so she has even more work to do when she gets home. She is trapped. This woman may suffer fatigue."

If you're stuck in that kind of situation, may be it seems like there's nothing you can do. But according to Dr. Alpern, the symptoms of fatigue associated with stress can often be alleviated by doing the following:

- Practise relaxation techniques. They make take only 10 or 15 minutes to learn.
- Once you know the techniques, use them to take a couple of 10 or 15-minute "vacations" from your work around the home or office every day. "Doing these exercises and paying attention to your feelings can break that all-day feeling of tension," says Dr. Alpern.

Anaemia

Take the iron out of a bridge, and it'll collapse. Run low on iron in your blood, and may be you'll collapse. Iron deficiency can lead to fatigue.

Even if our diet is iron-rich, we might have trouble holding onto it. In women, heavy menstrual flow may deplete the body's stores of iron resulting in frequent fatigue, says James D. Cook, M.D. head of the division of hematology at the University of Kansas Medical Center. Men, on the other hand, may suffer from iron deficiency due to gastrointestinal bleeding. Such bleeding might be virtually unnoticeable yet sufficient to cause anaemia.

Pregnant women and children going through rapid growth periods often need more iron than the rest of us. If this need is not met, they too may have iron-deficiency anaemia and that washed-out feeling.

The Recommended Daily Allowance for adults and children over four years of age is 18 milligrams. Among the best food sources of iron are liver, lean ground meat, beans, apples and spinach. Iron in large amounts can be harmful, however.

Diabetes

Chronic weariness, along with thirst and general weakness, can signify the onset of diabetes. Nonstop fatigue might also be the first sign of hepatitis, a thyroid disorder, mononucleosis, tuberculosis or infection.

"More often than not, emotional factors of stress or depression are the cause of fatigue," says Dr. Alpern. But if you do feel tired all the time, even right after you get up in the morning, call your doctor for a check-up.

Heart Disease

One of the first warning signs of heart disease—and, occasionally, the only signal—may be fatigue.

"The word 'fatigue', to a cardiologist, is very important," says Dr. Alpern. "Fatigue is one of the things we look for in the person in his 50s or 60s as a possible warning sign of an impending heart attack. Fatigue may be associated with a change in the heart, so it is good reason to go in for a check-up, particularly in the age group we're talking about."

What to do about fatigue, in this situation, may not be as simple. A heart problem, obviously, calls for immediate medical intervention. If you feel tired all the time, or if you have any other symptoms of heart attack, such as squeezing chest pain below the breast-bone, general weakness or nausea, seek medical help without delay.

Depression

Your only son is about to marry an intelligent, beautiful young woman. She's the kind of a person you would have picked yourself for someone as special as your boy. There's every reason for joy in your life, but that's not how you feel. You're very sad and very tired. And, suddenly, this wedding is becoming a problem.

"Fatigue often is a warning signal of a failure to master a problem," says Dr. Wharton. "Sometimes there is anticipation of a conflict, and other times the conflict is ongoing."

Another reason why a depressed person might feel exhausted is due to lack of sleep.

"Many depressed people may have serious trouble sleeping," says Dr. Wharton, "or they'll have recurring nightmares. The sleep disturbance is part of the depressive cycle. They'll wake up feeling tired. In fact, they've been sleeping but they've been having very troublesome dreams, which can be as exhausting as if they were struggling during the day, digging a ditch. They're digging a deeper and deeper hole, and never getting out of it. But you can start getting out of this hole if you begin to understand why you feel depressed. It's often possible to see what you can do to prevent trouble in the future, to prevent this fatigue reaction which makes everything an effort."

But there's more to getting better than recognizing what makes you depressed. Once you know the underlying cause of your emotional downturn, you then have to change the way you react to the situation or failing that change the situation. For either option, you might need the emotional help of a trained mental-health practitioner.

"Sometimes, getting better means taking a look at how you have dealt with crises in the past and learning ways to deal with new crises," says Dr. Wharton. "Other times, it requires an exploration of one's whole past. But the good news is that fatigue of this sort is usually treatable."

Whatever the cause of your fatigue, it's important to obtain an expert diagnosis. Your weariness could be the result of simple muscle fatigue, stress, lack of exercise, or, says Dr. Alpern, "just about any disease the body could get, from a cold to the worst." Fortunately, most fatigue is not serious.

But are you really tired? Not just in need of a couple of early nights to put you back in fighting form but really bone tired. Waking up tired, too tired to make love, read a book, or go out and visit friends.

If so, you could be a victim of what doctors are calling the Plague of the Age-chronic fatigue.

Tiredness, they say, cripples more people's lives than that renowned ABC of scourges—arthritis, bronchitis and chronic heart disease.

But why is it that some people are permanently exhausted without making excessive physical or mental effort, while others are brimming over with vim and vigour?

The answer lies less in their genes than in their lifestyles.

Here are 10 tips to beat the fatigue barrier.

- **Travel light.** You cannot be fit and fat. Exceed your correct weight by only 10 percent and you are twice as likely to have symptoms of chronic illness.
- **Don't spare your legs.** The toll-tale symptoms of fatigue—pain, tiredness and aching—are most commonly experienced in the legs.

  But stamina comes from using your muscle power. Do conditioning leg exercises or try to take a regular 30-minute daily walk.
- **Keep in the pink.** Generally, your skin will be pink if your blood is rich and red. Red is the colour of the vital oxygen-carrying pigment of the blood, and red blood cells are nourished by iron.

  Eat a weekly meal of liver, three or four slices of wholemeal bread a day, some dried fruit and nuts, and generous helpings of beans and green leafy vegetables.
- **Be temperate with sweets.** Go easy on the sugar. Best of all, cut it out. Eat instead unrefined carbohydrates such as bread, potatoes and rice. The body breaks them down into glucose. Make your meals small and regular. Always have a proper breakfast.
- **Get your sleep pattern right.** Sleep as and when you need to. Take catnaps. Don't be a 'sleep cheat', making inroads on the hours of rest your body needs by staying up late.
- Avoid the 'indoor climate syndrome.' Tiredness, together with smarting eyes, headaches and increased irritability, can all be part of this.

  Overcome it by making sure of an equable temperature, adequate ventilation, comfortable humidity and air free from noxious chemicals, gases and dust.

- **Check your fitness.** Fatigue can be the result of chronic infection—such as ascystitis, gum disease or sinusitis. Or of the pain drain. Never be content to endure chronic pain or feeling below par.

  Pain is a warning signal that something needs looking into.

- Make sure you are not allergic. Fatigue may be caused by your body's constant exposure to substances to which it is allergic or hypersensitive. They cover a wide spectrum ranging from Chinese food to knicker elastic and even mothers-in-law!

  You must try to identify these with the help of your doctor and eliminate them from your diet or environment.

- **Define your goals.** It is wonderful how you can overcome tiredness and generate vitality and drive if you concentrate your life force on clearly defined goals.

  Don't dwell on past failures, or be anxious about the future. Devote your energies to living in the here-and-now.

- **Mobilise your latent powers.** Each night as you go to bed, and each morning as you wake, lie back with your eyes closed and in a state of maximum relaxation.

  Whisper to your subconscious mind: "Each day I'm getting stronger. My stores of energy are growing. I have the power to conquer fatigue."

  And that is a prescription which, if conscientiously followed, can transform your life.

Natural Healing Practices

Within each one of us there lies a "healing system" capable of fighting off disease, combating infection and bringing us greater energy, vitality, and well-being. In any medical text we can read about the digestive system, the circulatory system, or the "nervous system", but nowhere can we find a chapter on the healing system. Yet it is this very "healing system" which allows all our other "systems" to function with brilliant precision. Our healing system is the organizing force through which all our body systems function with a deep intelligence and miraculous sense of balance and wholeness.

Bernie Siegel, M.D., the famous Yale surgeon and author, speaks of this healing system eloquently when he says "As a surgeon, I cut into the body and I rely on it to heal. I don't have to yell into the wound and tell it how to heal." The body, in its own infinite wisdom, knows how to heal. The healing system lies within us. Our body has its own natural ability to heal. Though in certain situations, surgery or drugs may be life saving, it is our internal healing system which allows ultimate life. We all know of patients who have lost the "will to live." No matter how valiant the efforts of medical experts, how advanced the technologies, how genuine the prayers of friends and relatives, these patients will continue on a downhill course, until and unless they find within themselves some sense of meaning with which to embrace life and connect to something greater than themselves, something greater than their sense of illness or despair. It is this "will to live", to prosper, to grow, to contribute, to engage life with passionate involvement, which most directly contributes to the overall health of our healing system.

"Healing" comes from the root word, "whole", to be one. In searching out our own individual path for health and healing, we will inevitably embark on a journey that leads us into our own sense of wholeness, uniqueness and self-discovery. It is important to understand that no two patients are alike. In fact, two patients with the "same" diagnosis of migraine headaches will, in most cases, require two completely different treatments, based on their own unique stresses, genetic background and lifestyle choices. So, in reality, two "cases" of migraine are two different diseases. Healing, in its essence, is an adventure in self-discovery.

New Realities: New Capacities

One of the greatest discoveries of the human potential movement is that as new realities are demonstrated, new capacities come into being. How many today remember Roger Bannister? He was an Oxford medical student who was the first person to run the mile in under four minutes. He broke the "four-minute barrier." Until that time, it was believed that no human could break that barrier. No such reality was ever demonstrated. Now the most fascinating part of the story is that within 46 days of Bannister's breakthrough, John Landing broke the four-minute mile. And now, at this time, literally thousands of runners have broken the four-minute barrier. So we see that as new realities are demonstrated, new capacities come into being.

The challenge for all of us is to open ourselves to the "new realities" that have been demonstrated through recent advances in mind/body, medicine and psychoneuroimmunology. These new medical disciplines are beginning to detail the many ways in which our thoughts, our feelings, our psychological and spiritual beliefs affect our physical health. By recognizing these "new realities" of what is possible, we can begin to develop "new capacities" for health, healing and greater well-being. These new capacities can help us access our own healing systems. Here is a story that Rachel Naomi Remen, M.D., a physician and healer in northern California, tells. This is the story of the acorn. For one moment, imagine an acorn trying to make sense of itself, trying to understand itself, by describing itself. It might say "I'm about 1 inch long, flat on one side, pointed on the other, brown in colour, hard to the touch, etc. etc." But this description fails to capture the true essence of the acorn. "It's important to realize", Dr. Remen says, "that an acorn cannot make sense of itself without knowing about the oak tree and without knowing that deep inside of itself, there is a mechanism waiting to unfold which knows exactly how to become that fullness of expression" of the oak tree. She says "there is an impulse, a yearning in each one of us, towards our own wholeness", our own fullness of expression. It is this impulse, this yearning towards our own wholeness which leads us into the healing process.

We can access our healing system, and begin the adventure into self-discovery and wholeness, allowing us to fully realize our capacities for health, healing and a sense of well-being.

According to Harold Koenig, M.D., the author of **The Healing Power of Faith,** healing can include dramatic, sudden physical cures, but is not confined to the 'miraculous' or the spectacular. Perhaps for most people, the healing power of faith involves a healing of the mind and emotions, the intangible spirit, and of relationships with others.

Faith can put physical illness beneath us, where it belongs, return dominion to us, and give us power to live victorious and fulfilling lives. People who regularly attend religious service and pray individually are 40% less likely to have diastolic hypertension than those who seldom participate in these religious activities.

People who attend religious services regularly may have stronger immune systems than their less religious counterparts. Those who never or rarely attend such services tend to have the highest levels of Interleukin-6, perhaps indicating a weakened or overactive immune system.

People who attend religious services regularly are hospitalized less often and leave the hospital sooner than people who never or rarely participate in such services. The deeper a person's religious faith, the less likely he or she is to be crippled by depression during and after hospitalization for physical illness.

Religious people have healthier lifestyles, according to one study. Such people have about 1/3 the rate of alcohol abuse and are about 1/3 as likely to smoke as those who seldom participate in congregational worship.

Religious youth show significantly lower levels of drug and alcohol abuse, premature sexual involvement, and criminal delinquency than their non-religious peers. They are also less likely to express suicidal thoughts or make actual attempts on their lives.

Elderly people with a deep, personal religious faith have a stronger sense of well-being and life satisfaction than their less religious peers. Religious people live longer and physically healtheir lives than their non-religious counterparts.

There are ways to increase your healing ability, according to researcher Marie T. Russell. In her view, everyone is a healer. Just as everyone is alive and breathing, everyone has the power and the ability to connect with the life energy that brings in healing. You don't need training, though you can certainly learn techniques and earn confidence by taking classes; you don't need certification, though if you're going to become a "healer" officially and provide your services for hire, then certification is recommended. But, if you're wanting to increase your healing ability so that you can use it for your own healing, then it's right there waiting for you to tap into it.

Many of us go through life seeking healing from other people when really the only person who can heal us is ourselves. We run to doctors or healers to have them "heal" us. Yet, the body is the one which heals itself with the assistance of whatever remedies or assistance it receives. Whether one is taking pills, vitamins, or herbs, the body is the one that utilizes these as it sees fit. You could be eating the best foods, yet your body has to know and be capable of utilizing them in order for you to be "healed."

The body is the one which knows what to do with the calcium, the vitamins, the enzymes, the healing energy... If it didn't have its own innate intelligence, it would not know how to utilize these healing substances that we ingest and accept into our being. The medicines or the medical staff are not the healers... the body itself is the healer. Thus, the responsibility for healing oneself returns to its only true home, yourself. Possibly, you have felt helpless in healing yourself and you don't feel like you know where to start. A good place to start is with convincing yourself that you indeed can heal yourself. This means reprogramming the thoughts you carry. You might begin the re-programming with statements such as these:

My body is healing itself and the cells of my body are constantly "giving birth" to new healthy cells.

Everyday, I get healtheir and happier (and whatever other qualifications you want to increase in your life).

My body is constantly healing itself everyday and every moment.

Every little cell in my body is happy; every little cell in my body is well.

I am connected with the life force and always have enough energy and vitality to be completely healthy and happy.

Practise talking to yourself. (No, they won't lock you up.) If you are afraid of being thought weird, speak silently to yourself... Talk to the cells of your body. Tell them you love them. Tell them you now give them permission to be healthy. Visualize (a fancy word for imagine) them being healthy and vibrant with life force. See your body being filled with radiant healing energy. Feel it spreading from the top of your head down to the bottom of your feet. Tell yourself that you now give yourself complete permission to be 100% healthy and 100% happy.

How to do Hands-on Self-healing

You can do "hands-on" healing on yourself. All you need is the willingness to accept that this is indeed possible and to give permission to have Divine energy flow through you.

Start by asking for Divine protection and see yourself surrounded by white light. A good way to do this is to fill your heart with light and then have the light keep expanding until you are filled with white light, and surrounded with light in a somewhat egg-shape. Hold up your left hand, palm outward, and ask for healing energy to flow through you. Imagine the healing energy coming in to your body through the palm of your left hand. You can visualize it as white light, or green energy, or whatever seems appropriate to you at the moment. Trust your intuition or gut feeling on this one, as different healing situations will call for different energies, or colours of light, or warmth, etc.

As you keep holding up your left hand and allowing the Divine energy to enter, place your right hand, palm down, on the area of your body which needs healing. You may feel some warmth entering your left hand, and the palm of your right hand may get hot. You might also feel a tingling or vibrating effect. This is the energy of healing moving through you. (If you don't feel anything, don't worry. The energy is still there—you simply are not sensitive to it yet.)

Relax and be grateful for the ability to be a channel for this energy. You may use this for digestion problems, muscle soreness, tense shoulders, headaches, stress, etc.

You may also use this God-given talent to share with friends. Teach them to connect with this force. Everyone is a healer. The body was built as a self-healing mechanism. When given the chance the body heals itself. Animals know this which is why they go off by themselves to rest when hurt or ill. The human animal (that's us) can also do the same. We can respect the needs of our body for quiet, rest, fasting, and healing energy. Listen to the quiet inner voice which guides you as to what you need to do. When feeling ill you may choose to take some time to be alone and quietly apply some healing energy to your body. After all, this body is the only one you have got. When it is properly connected to life energy it can heal itself, so plug in to the source and heal thyself...

If you are dealing with a disease or chronic illness, says Dr. Judith Orloff, MD, you'll have many decisions to make regarding your options for care. Should you undergo open heart surgery, medication or meditation? Whatever condition or disease you are dealing with, your intuition can be a valuable tool in deciding what treatment is right for you. But how can you quiet the hubbub of well-meaning voices (physicians, family, friends, even your manicurist) that threaten to drown out the voice of your intuition? As illustrated in the book, Dr. Judith Orloff's Guide to Intuitive Healing, the following five tactics can help you access that unbiased inner authority, your intuition.

Notice Your Beliefs

Does this sound familiar? "What did I do wrong? Why me? It's hopeless. It's unfair. I'm a victim." If so, you've got to change your mindset, or your internalized belief system, and put it to work, so it is healing, not harmful. When you hear these negative voices, say, "Thanks for sharing," and move on.

In all types of illness, from cancer to a cold, never fail to remember the mind's capacity to heal, even what has been deemed "unhealable." By lovingly learning to refocus your intuition, you can strive to cure or at least improve any health situation.

The following exercise can help you articulate your beliefs about healing and illness, and, if necessary, can help you change them. Ask yourself:

- Do your beliefs give you strength during illness? If not, are you ready to find ones that do?
- In a health crisis, what role does your intuition play? How far would you trust it?
- How do you treat yourself when you're sick or in pain? If you're self-critical, how can you turn this into self-compassion?
- Do you believe love can heal? How about humour? Are you willing to put them to the test?

Be in Your Body

Our tendency, once we feel pain or get sick, is to check out of our bodies ("That's it, I'm outta here.") But to do so is to ignore two intuitive truths. Intuitive Truth number one is that the more love and consciousness you bring to your body, the better chance you'll have of mending it. Intuitive Truth number two says that if you resist discomfort, it will persist. But if you soften around it, it will lessen.

When you are in tune with your body, there's no guarantee that your pain will miraculously dissipate, though it might. What will happen, however, is that you will enter into a relationship with a force that can provide clues on how to heal. This is a very different philosophy from just swallowing a pill, sitting back, and waiting for the pain to go away.

The following Meditation for Dealing with Pain and Illness can help you access the healing powers that come from paying attention to your body:

1. Relax into the discomfort. Simply let the pain be.

2. Intuitively tune into the discomfort. Does it have a colour? Texture? Temperature? Ask the discomfort: What can I learn from you. How can I ease my pain?
3. Feel your discomfort completely. As you inhale, breathe in all your pain. Visualize it as a cloud of dark smoke. Now picture the dark smoke being purified by your reserves of love and compassion. Exhale, letting the dark smoke flow out of your body in the form of clear white light.

Sense Your Body's Subtle Energy

Never underestimate your energy's ability to ease suffering, accelerate healing, or even cure disease. Our bodies are composed of energy centres known as chakras. For the purposes of the following meditation, we'll focus on the heart chakra, the main generator that fuels our healing system. The heart chakra is located in the middle of your chest, over the diaphragm. To activate it, try the Meditation for Opening the Heart:

1. Get very quiet. Relax your body and focus on your breathing. Gently place your hand over your heart chakra, and hold it there. Now get ready to visualize.
2. Concentrate on a person, place, or animal that you really love. Focus on feeling love, and notice how its energy equivalent localizes in your mid-chest.
3. Pay attention to sensations such as warmth, cold, or tingling in your heart chakra. As you practise, a vortex of positive energy in your heart chakra will get built. This is the hub of your healing. During times of pain or illness, tap into it.

You may also find it useful to practise sharing energy with a friend. To do so, place your hands over a friend's chest. Focus on feeling your heart chakra opening. Spend a few minutes allowing love to go freely from your heart, down to your arms, out of your palms, and into your friend. Then reverse roles. You'll discover that love nourishes you as much as it does the person you're healing.

Ask for Inner Guidance

When you have a diagnosis and are ready to make treatment decisions, gather as much information as you can about your illness, but don't stop there. Take all the time you need to listen intuitively. No matter how impressive the scientific evidence, your choice must sit well with you. Asking yourself the following questions can help you access your intuition as you make these important decisions:

- What does my gut say? Is it tied in knots or relaxed? Does an option feel "right" or "off"?
- Do I sleep better or worse at night thinking about a particular approach? Does going ahead with it make me feel more at peace?
- When I quietly tune in, what images or impressions come to me? Are they telling me to go ahead? Wait? Seek out another alternative? Pose specific questions to your intuition. Evaluate the response.

Listen to Your Dreams

In our world, science's vigilant effort to quantify illness could profit by collaborating with dreams. Relegating hard science to one camp and visionary dreams to another is a no-win proposition for everyone. The two can work together. Dreaming is hinged on the surrender of our thinking minds. More healing is possible without our ordinary walls intact when creativity is at its peak. Healing equals Creativity. In terms of your body, dreams offer brilliant solutions to health issues that may have never dawned on you before. There are indications of whether a healing dream is intuitively accurate. The following are tried-and-true touchstones:

- Exceptionally vibrant imagery, colours or sounds
- An oddly impersonal tone, neutrally imparting information
- A sense of indisputable "knowing:" in your body
- A crispness and clarity to segments

The following Four Tips on Intuitive Dream interpretations can help you get the most out of your dreams:

1. On awakening, record your dream immediately in a journal.
2. Notice those images and dream symbols to which you're especially drawn or those that move you.
3. As soon as possible, go into meditation. Hold the symbol in your mind. Specifically ask to be shown its significance.

4. Pay particular attention to any images, scenarios, memories, or physical sensations that arise. These intuitions come from the deepest part of you. They will explain your symbol.

Anti-oxidants Slow Down Aging Process

In a study published in American Journal of Physiology, Christian Lecawenburgh, a professor in UF's College of Health and Human Performance, found that anti-oxidant intervention, which can come from taking vitamin supplements or from a steady routine of exercise, slows parts of the aging process.

"Our most significant finding was that anti-oxidant intervention slows down basal skeletal muscle oxidation, which causes the body to age," says Leeuwenburgh, who did the study with researchers from the Washington University School of Medicine. "This is the first evidence of this."

Aging and Tissue and Muscle Loss

Regular exercise or a diet including plenty of anti-oxidants such as vitamin E, vitamin C and Beta carotene, all of which fight the tendency of oxygen to slowly break down muscle mass, might protect against the type of tissue and muscle loss that occur as individuals grow older, Leeuwenburgh says.

"We were surprised to see that regular exercise training was about as effective in reducing levels of oxidation as a diet of anti-oxidants," Leeuwenburgh says. "The combined effect of anti-oxidants and exercise, however, didn't cause a significantly lower level of muscle oxidation, which was interesting." The study also was the first of its kind to show that levels of oxidation in the body can be determined noninvasively, by using specific markers in the urine.

Aging and Heart Disease

Leeuwenburgh recommends daily anti-oxidant intake, especially vitamin E, because it also has been proven to protect against heart disease. Exercising more and eating less also will help people live longer, he says.

Natural Slimming

Going on a diet is like officially declaring war—you have to be prepared for a long siege, on short rations, a high level of public interest and the risk of failure! Like any battle, you'll need a plan of action, so here is a strategy for a different way to fight those extra kilos.

1. Cover the very worst photograph of yourself in clear plastic and stick it inside the refrigerator so that it is the first and last thing you see every time you open the door.
2. Give yourself a cut-off time for eating: resolve to never eat after 8 pm.
3. Put rings on a finger of each hand. Stare at the left-hand ring and think of everything you hate about being fat—how your thighs rub together when you walk, how your clothes look like sofa covers and how you gasp when bending to tie your laces. Then stare at the right hand ring and visualise yourself in your ideal size easy-moving and elegant in new clothes.

   Do this often enough to imprint the two images in your mind. It will be harder for your hands to add forbidden kilos when they are constantly reminding you of what you're trying to leave behind.
4. Eliminate the word 'cheat' from your vocabulary. Give yourself permission for an occasional bite of something marvellous and then enjoy it thoroughly.
5. Never go into a food store when you are hungry.
6. If you feel you can't live without something to nibble, try toasted pumpkin seeds. They need to be shelled, which is a cumbersome work, so fewer of them are eaten. Peanuts in their shells also slow down the eating process.
7. Curd mustard makes an excellent substitute for mayonnaise.

8. Stick to the edges of the market, where fresh fruit and vegetables, chicken and dairy products are usually to be found. Especially avoid the soft drink and cake shops. If it is necessary to pass the cake shops, close your eyes.
9. You don't have to stick to three meals a day. Divide your daily ration into a number of smaller meals. But nominate eating times and then stick to them.
10. Learn to like drinking water. Chill a two litre container, squeeze half a lemon into it and drop in some of the rind for extra flavour. If your tap water is really horrible, consider investing in a filter. Aim at drinking at least six large glasses a day and always drink one before a meal.
11. If you really crave for something sweet to drink, why not slowly eat a slice of watermelon instead?
12. Save half the calories of butter by blending it with an equal quantity of curd.
13. Take your own lunch to work. Buy a special plastic container in which you can pre-make a pretty looking salad with lots of interesting vegetables and a small portion of lean meat or fish. If you have no time in the morning, make brown bread sandwiches. As many fillings can be frozen, some sandwiches can be made at the weekend for the days ahead.
14. Avoid fast foods.
15. Walk tall, stand tall and sit tall. This kind of passive exercise opens up your rib-cage and allows the oxygen to flow in better-and it is oxygen that burns up fat. A simple trick for perfect posture is to keep your knee caps up when you stand or walk. "Think" your neck longer by imagining that a thread is attached to the top of your head, suspending you from the sky.
16. Give yourself an attainable goal every day and keep a list of your successes. Goals can include having a totally sugar-free day (which means not even one biscuit or a totally chocolate-free day) or a 30-minute walk.
17. Grill meat much longer than you usually do because this melts out the fat. Then, before putting the meat on a plate stand it on a paper napkin a minute. Every calorie counts!

18. Feed your freezer.... let it gobble up left-overs so you're not tempted to finish them. Freeze one-serve portions of your own special, slimming meals. For instance, a chicken steamed over an aromatic mixture of herbs and vegetables and then broken into pieces can become the main component of quite a few low-calorie meals.
19. Make careful lists and then shop for food only once a week or even less if possible. Aim to carry the parcels yourself. You'll think twice about heavy bottles of juice and litres of ice-cream if you know you're going to lug them home.
20. Try to go vegetarian at least thrice a week. When you do, make a really luscious meal. You might get hooked.
21. When you go out to lunch order fresh carrot juice with your meal. It is so delicious that it justifies investing in a juicer.
22. Limit your shopping choices to foods containing less than 30 per cent fat. This means no more cold meats, cheese or potato crisps.
23. If you crave for sweetness, carry artificial sweetners wherever you go, so that the invitation to a cup of tea at a friend's house does not lead to an arm-wrestle with the sugar bowl.
24. Keep the most dangerous of your favourite snacks in the freezer. If you have to wait for something to thaw you may change your mind about having it. Don't let the children nag you into leaving the biscuits and chocolate at room-temperature—teach them to be patient too. Better still encourage children to eat fruit, toast or gheeless or oilless chapatis as a snack.
25. Eat slowly. The brain has an "I'm full" mechanism, which usually comes into effect after about 15 minutes of eating. Yours might have been reduced to a whisper after years of being ignored, so encourage it to speak up again. Plan to spend at least 20 minutes eating, chewing slowly and putting your knife and fork down between mouthfuls.
26. If you were told as a child that it was good to clean your plate, tell yourself that now you're grownup. It is polite to leave a little something to show the world you've had enough. This will cause a lot of internal argument—a good test for your developing will power.

27. When you feel desperate to put something in your mouth, try cleaning your teeth. If that doesn't help, sugarless chewing gum might.
28. Stick a photograph of someone whose figure you admire, up on the bathroom mirror. Think of it as the "future you." Do a visualisation every morning and before going to bed at night.
29. Try weak, black tea instead of having it with milk and sugar. If the taste is too terrible to bear, experiment with herb teas—some of these have really interesting flavours which can distract your anguished tastebuds.
30. Don't taste while cooking; rely on your experience, a good recipe book or the taste of another palate.
31. Develop food consciousness. Don't be food obsessive, though. A food-conscious person is aware of calorie values and nutrients and does not eat mindlessly. A person obsessed with food is liable to eat faddily or binge-and-starve.
32. Do something you've been putting off: one of the main causes of depression, say experts, is what they term "delay in taking constructive action." When we're feeling down, many of us turn to food for comfort. So write that letter, make that phone call, clean the stove... do whatever you've been feeling guilty about not doing and beat those fattening blues.
33. An active shopping trip can burn off calories, but concentrate on running around after clothes or homeware and steer clear of food shops.
34. Take the salt cellar off the table and don't use any while cooking. You will be surprised at how quickly you learn to prefer the flavour. Salt causes the body to retain water which makes you look and feel heavy.
35. Make yourself some healthy treats like sliced carrots, celery and capsicum. Keep these standing in iced water in the refrigerator—they make delicious, crunchy, low calorie snacks.
36. Walk the dog, preferably a young dog which is sure to take you on a brisker hike than you might otherwise contemplate. If you don't own one, borrow one-your neighbour could be very grateful.
37. Use grated cheese, which is better than chunks of it. And to

stop you overindulging your 'cheese tooth', on chunks that can vary with the slip of a knife, buy small packets rather than tins.

38. Remember that one level teaspoonful of sugar contains 70 calories.
39. Don't deny yourself favourite foods but find new ways to prepare them. For instance don't cut roasting potatoes—use them whole, so that there is less surface to absorb fat. Or bake them on the oven shelf and avoid all fat.
40. If you think you're being virtuous by using margarine instead of butter, forget it! They're both 740 calories per level tablespoonful (or 20g).
41. Try walking for 20 to 30 minutes every day. If you use public transport, get off a stop or two earlier each day until you've established a good daily hike.
42. Eating out? Cut out on starchy and oily items... Avoid cream on your dessert and in your coffee (about 450 calories a dollop). Cheese and biscuits could cost you 1,500 calories.
43. Use your loaf! Crusty bread from the bakery has about the same calories per slice as sliced bread but you are likely to cut yourself thicker slices. Wherever you buy your bread, make sure it's wholemeal or wholegrain—apart from the fact that it is much more nourishing, it also provides valuable fibre. Bread has fewer calories than biscuits or pies. Oil free chapatis are best of all.
44. If you're making sandwiches, avoid spreading butter or margarine on the bread. Instead, use moist fillings such as egg mashed with a little non-fat curd or cucumber on low calorie homemade cheese. Or use a lettuce or spinach leaf as one half of the sandwich.
45. Collect gourmet vinegars. Make your own by adding fresh parsley leaves to good quality white vinegar. Use them without oil on salads or in marinades.
46. Every time you reach a goal, reward yourself with something that is not food oriented, like a facial or a new pair of ear-rings or the latest ghazal cassette. Tell yourself that you deserve to be pampered this way.

47. Look into everyone else's shopping bags and notice how little fresh food and how absolute junk they're eating. Imagine you are being complimented on the wisdom of your own choices.
48. Buy opaque containers for the refrigerator so that you don't look delicious things in the eye.
49. If you are invited to a dinner party, take along the gift of a special dish that also just happens to be on your new eating plan.
50. Try to organise parties at your own house so that you are in control of what is served.
51. Don't exercise alone if you have kids—they will love joining you in the one-two and one-two routine. Watch TV while you work out, jump on a minitrampoline or ride an exercise bike.
52. If you must eat pancakes, use whole wheat flour with vegetable concentrate.
53. Buy one beautiful outfit in the size you're aiming to be and hang it in the wardrobe. Take it out often, hold it up in front of the mirror and visualise yourself looking wonderful in it.
54. When it rains and you can't walk home, hike around the shopping centre. Go up and down the stairs rather than in the lift. Good for making your calf muscles curvy and sexy.
55. One orange takes longer to eat and is more satisfying than the two or three oranges that go into a glass of juice.
56. If you really crave dessert buy a one portion pack as an occasional treat. Then you can't have seconds!
57. Popcorn is very satisfying to chew and is low in calories and high in fibre.
58. Think of yourself as a person with energy. Buy running shoes and a headphone tape player—it will make you feel like a dancer or an athlete when you exercise.
59. Don't cut yourself off from the sensual pleasure and creativity of food. Join a cooking class. Try cuisines that are low in calories and high in flavour.
60. In restaurants, don't even look at the dessert list.
61. If your personal reward system includes the occasional beer, split a bottle with a friend.

62. Next time you feel like a snack, pick up some dumb-bells or a couple of books (this is where last year's telephone books can come handy). Stand in front of the mirror and do some lifting exercises over your head. Exercise is a mood elevator as well as a muscle trimmer.

63. When you're sick and tired of steamed or grilled food, use a paper towel to rub a few drops of oil onto a non-stick pan, then, saute or stir-fry food in its own juices. Or use a pan liner.

64. Wear tight fitting clothes or a belt when you go out to dinner—it will help you get the "I'm full" signal sooner.

65. If you spend a lot of time sitting in a car or at a desk, grip the steering wheel or the desk-edge, straighten your arms and push back as hard as you can—often. This will help strengthen your back muscles.

66. Take up gardening. All that digging, bending, tending and weeding is good for you, and the rewards of perfect blooms, tangy herbs and fresh vegetables are a bonus.

67. Keep the salt and sugar containers somewhere difficult to reach or remember, like a high cupboard.

68. Slice cucumber, stir oatmeal into a thick paste with water... This recipe is not for eating but for treating yourself. Cover your face with the oat paste and your eyelids with the cucumber, then lie down and think of yourself as a beautiful person under your home facial.

69. While you are resting, press your legs hard against the sides. Repeat with your arms and legs together. Then relax again—dieters deserve some indulgence time too.

70. When you dry yourself after a bath, be brisk about it—wiggle and twist against the towel. Massage yourself with lotion until you tingle and smell marvellous.

71. Never tell anyone that dieting is difficult—misery loves company. If you feel depression creeping up, do the thing you least feel like doing—washing the windows, writing up your tax figures or cleaning out the kitchen cupboards, for instance. The sense of virtue will instantly kill the blues.

72. Never lose an opportunity to exercise your muscles. While

sitting, talking on the phone, flex your buttocks so that you rise slightly in the seat. Hold for a few seconds before relaxing. When you've rung off, stick your tongue out as far as you can and then try to touch your nose with it. This is good for singling double chins.

73. At home use a smaller plate than usual for your meals so that they don't look pathetic, rattling around in the middle of a big dish.

74. Which cereal? Calorie-wise they don't vary that much, averaging about 400 cals per 30 g serve. But it is very easy to get 60g of channa (gram) which is a very heavy cereal, whereas you can fill the bowl with puffed wheat and find you've eaten only 270 kg. Porridge made with hot water rather than milk is satisfying too.

75. Put extra energy into the housework. Cleaning, making beds and vacuuming all consume about 15 cals a minute.

76. If you drop something, keep your legs straight and bend from the waist to pick it up—provided that it is something very light, of course. Anything heavy could put your back out.

77. Have a large glass of mineral water just before you go out to dinner.

78. Don't weigh yourself more than once a week. If you are disappointed with the results, check your own biological clock; the chances are you're premenstrual and therefore carrying temporary excess fluid.

79. Make sure to see your doctor regularly while you're dieting. Apart from the fact that your heart and blood pressure should be monitored, it is good to have professional approval of your progress.

80. Put a cushion or book between your knees when you're sitting and then squeeze them together tightly and often to trim down thigh flab.

81. Work out a put-it-on put-it-off chart for small treats. An average biscuit is worth about 250 calories, so burn it off with 12 minutes of brisk walking or gardening, seven minutes of walking up and down stairs or 12 minutes of disco dancing. A half hour run is worth seven biscuits.

82. Decorate a room. All that stretching and bending burns calories and keeps you supple and you won't be able to snack with your hands covered in paint or paste.

83. Switch to skim milk and save 880 cals per 600 ml without losing the nutrients.

84. Measure your daily milk allowance into your own, special container. Then you'll know how much there is left at any time. An extra half cup is worth 360 cals.

85. Eat most of your day's calories early in the day, to give your digestion plenty of time to process the food. Then you will sleep better at night.

86. Fill your weekends with activities that are action not food-oriented.

87. If you have trouble slowing down your eating, use chopsticks instead of a knife and folks. Or try switching cutlery to the 'wrong' hands.

88. Whip non-fat home made cheese and curd together in the blender. Eat flavoured herbs or garlic.

89. Skimmed milk and dissolved gelatin will whip into dessert topping. Sweeten it lightly with an artificial sweetner.

90. Make sure you get plenty of sleep-that is when your body restores itself, and if you're losing weight there's a lot of restoration to be done.

91. If you crave ice-cream, try a skim-milk variety or buy a single cone.

92. When someone or something makes you cross or sad, tell a sympathetic friend or write it all down in a letter or a diary. Just don't brood-there's nothing that leads you to the cake tin faster than self-pity or self-reproach.

93. Make an appointment with the very best hairdresser in town. Even if you have to save up, have the best perm, cut and colour you can. This is an important step to becoming the new you—your friends and relations will be full of praise.

94. If you have had a bad day and blow your diet, don't panic. Remember, nobody's perfect. Instead of criticising yourself for one day's failure, praise yourself for all the successful

days that preceded it and all the even more successful ones that will follow.

95. Never waste a moment to tighten muscles. Even when you're sitting in an armchair, you can straighten your back, rest your arms along its arms, grasp a cushion between your feet and raise and lower it. Bend your knees towards your chest, hold for the count of five and slowly straighten them. Both these exercises are great for leg and abdomen muscles.

96. As an aid to eating slowly, substitute potatoes with brown rice, or cut them up into very small dice and then eat them without the aid of the knife. You'll spend at least as much time pushing them around with a fork as eating them.

97. Take up a new hobby. It is hard to snack while playing the sitar or playing tennis. Sewing, knitting or embroidery are fiddly occupations too, with which coffee cups and food crumbs do not readily mix.

98. Write these tips on a paper and stick or pin some of them to various places you look at often—the bathroom mirror, the kitchen noticeboard, your desk—then make them part of your life. When you have, add new ones.

99. Fall in love with your partner all over again—the chances are you won't eat a thing!

100. Learn yoga asanas from a book or attend yoga classes.

Now we demonstrate to you the imaginary body technique of maintaining ideal weight. If possible do this exercise along with friends who also wish to slim down, put on weight if they are too thin, or otherwise wish to attain ideal body weight and body shape.

Here is the exercise: Stay away from disturbance for half-an-hour. Stand comfortably barefoot. Your body relaxed and your eyes closed. Breathe regularly but naturally, not deeply. Count one when you breathe in, and two when you breathe out. Do this for a few minutes till your breathing is regular.

Balance your weight evenly on both feet. Feel the sensation of your feet on the ground. Run your attention of your whole body, slowly, picking up any sensations that you feel and relaxing any areas that feel tense.

In this exercise, we will distinguish your real body, and your imaginary body which you picture in your mind. Raise your **real** right arm. Extend it, sensing the sensations in the muscles all over your body. Feel the sensations in your fingers, palm, arm, shoulder, chest. Lower your arm picking up all the sensations that arise from this movement.

Raise and lower your right arm several times, picking up all the muscular sensations as they arise. Do so now.

Now, visualise your right arm in your mind, with all the sensations that you can imagine. Raise this imaginary arm, trying to experience it as clearly as possible. Lower this imaginary arm, again trying to feel the movement as intensely as you can. Now raise your **real** arm, then your imaginary **arm.** Alternate raising your real and imaginary right arms several times.

Repeat the procedure with your real left arm and imaginary left arm, trying to feel the imaginary arm as much as the real arm.

Rotate your shoulders and arms around their horizontal axis. Repeat with your imaginary shoulder and arms alternatively. Rotate your real shoulders and arms in the opposite direction. Repeat with your imaginary shoulders and arms alternatively.

Raise both your real arms over your head and clasp your hands. At the same time feel your imaginary arms and hands hanging by your sides (Pause).

Simultaneously but slowly **lower** your real arms, while **raising** your imaginary arms, trying to experience them as clearly as the real arms. Now lower your imaginary arms while raising your real arms. Repeat this procedure until you hardly distinguish between your real and imaginary arms.

Stand as before, eyes closed. With both legs jump as far as you can from where you are standing. Jump back. Do it again—forward. Again back. Again jump forward. Again jump back.

Now visualise your imaginary ideal body as you would like it to be as slim, trim and shapely. Make this imaginary body jump forward, exercising it as clearly and vividly as you can. Make your imaginary body jump back to where your real body is standing. Do this several times, with your imaginary body.

Now jump forward with your imaginary body. Now jump with your real body into your imaginary body. Feel the sensations all over your real body. Do you feel more than you used to?

Walk around and notice the difference in your earlier and present sensations. Open your eyes, and notice if you perceive things around you differently as well.

If you can, increase your awareness of your imaginary body by slowly rotating your real body in one direction and your imaginary body in the opposite direction. Reverse these directions several times.

Again stand up as before, relaxed and eyes closed. Sense the position and sensation of every part of your body from head to foot. How much of your feet touch the floor? Is your weight borne by your heels, or by the edges of your feet? How do your leg muscles feel? Sense and visualise every detail. Move up to your hips, buttocks, stomach. Sense their position, size, feel where is your fat concentrated. Now move to your chest, the back. Is there strain on the back? Do your shoulders ache? How do your arms feel. Move to your neck. Pick the sensations on it, as also its shape and weight. Feel the sensations on your face, nose, eyes. Visualise them vividly as they are. Move to your forehead and scalp. Notice the feel of your hair on the scalp, neck, forehead. Feel your ears and nose. Try to pick any sensation from these organs that you can get. How are they positioned with respect to your body? Sense all this and obtain a clear feel and image of your full body.

Now imagine as fully and clearly as you can— how you would like your body to be-slim-shapely, healthy. Take your own time to create in every detail your ideal body. Hold this image and breathe into it.

Now imagine your ideal body one foot in front of you, so you can see its back. Jump into your ideal body. How does it feel? If uncomfortable, jump out quickly. Adjust those parts or even whole image of your ideal body, so it is more realistic—and jump again into it. Repeat it until comfortable.

Begin to move around encased in your ideal body, allowing your experience of it to be integrated into your patterns of standing, walking, sitting and dancing.

According to psychologist Jean Houston "this exercise has been found particularly valuable for maintaining body weight at an optimal level. Suddenly and permanently the desire for sweets disappears, exercise routines are adopted and maintained. At the same time there is no sense of conscious effort or self-denial, those whose body is considerably larger than their ideal image often find that, for the moment at least they would not be truly comfortable by being 20 kilos thinner and are willing to make gradual changes in their body image, repeating this exercise over a period of months until they have achieved a body in which they feel truly at home."

Eat Well and Lose Weight

"Many years ago", says Suzanne Somers, author of **Eat Great and Lose Weight, "when I** was just starting out in television, I landed a guest-starring role on a hit series called Starsky and Hutch. Three days before I was supposed to start, I got a call from the producer. My ears perked up when I heard his voice. He told me that he and the director had been sitting around talking, and they decided I was just 'a little too chunky' for the part. They recast the role and I cried myself to sleep. I was twenty-nine years old and twenty pounds overweight. That's when my diet roller-coaster began. Determined to lose those pounds, I tried every diet in the world. The shakes, the calorie counting, the packaged foods, the fasting, the grapefruit, the cottage cheese, the celery... and guess what? They all worked. That's right. Every time I went on a diet, I lost weight. But, within a short time of going back to eating like a normal person, I would gain back all the weight and often a little extra. Then I'd scour the fashion magazines for the next dieting trend, and off I'd go on my path toward deprivation—all in the name of being thin.

"What I really wanted was to find a way to eat healthy, nutritious, yet flavourful foods in substantial portions and still lose weight. And I'm happy to tell you I have found it."

"After working with many nutritionists, reading books, and practising trial and error on my own body, I have finally found a way to control my weight without deprivation. I call my programme 'Somersizing,' and Somersizing is not a diet. Diet is a nasty four-letter word that conjures up negative thoughts of sacrifice and obsession and guilt. Based on eating everyday foods in specific combinations, Somersizing is a lifestyle that will change your way of thinking about how to lose weight and how to increase your energy. There are a few basic rules you will learn, and then you're free to eat whatever you want, in a restaurant, at home, or on the road."

"On the Somersize programme, you first eliminate a small group of what I call Funky Foods, foods that wreak havoc on our systems. Then you separate normal, everyday foods into four Somersize Food groups: proteins and fats, vegetables, carbohydrates, and fruits.

Finally, you follow these seven easy steps:

1. Eliminate all Funky Foods.
2. Eat Fruits alone, on an empty stomach.
3. Eat Proteins/Fats with Veggies.
4. Eat Carbos with Veggies and no fat.
5. Keep Proteins/Fats separate from Carbos.
6. Wait three hours between meals if switching from a Protein/ Fats meal to a Carbos meal, or vice versa.
7. Do not skip meals. Eat three meals a day and eat until you feel satisfied and comfortably full."

"Since I started properly combining my foods, "she goes on", I have trimmed down from 130 to 116 pounds—the amount I weighed as a teenager. And since I reached my goal weight, I have fluctuated no more than 3 pounds. I eat delicious foods—I eat cheese, I drink wine occasionally, and you would be shocked to know how much chocolate I eat and still maintain my weight."

"Some experts will argue that food-combining is a myth—a calorie is a calorie and it doesn't matter how you combine them, it only matters how many you eat and how many you burn off. The debate has gone on for many years, and I'm sure it will continue for many more. All I can tell you is that it works for me. I can eat all the wonderful foods I love and still lose weight. I don't have to give up flavour. I don't settle for boring meals with no sauce. I enjoy rich and flavourful foods. I don't count calories or fat grams", Somers concludes.

Physical Activity and Weight Control

How can physical activity help control your weight? Physical activity helps to control your weight by using excess calories that otherwise would be stored as fat. Your body weight is regulated by the number of calories you eat and use each day. Everything you eat contains calories, and everything you do uses calories, including sleeping, breathing, and digesting food. Any physical activity in addition to what you normally do will use extra calories.

Balancing the calories you use through physical activity with the calories you eat will help you achieve your desired weight. When you eat more calories than you need to perform your day's activities, your body stores the extra calories and you gain weight (a).

When you eat fewer calories than you use, your body uses the stored calories and you lose weight (b). When you eat the same amount of calories as your body uses, your weight stays the same (c).

Any type of physical activity you choose to do—strenuous activities such as running or aerobic dancing or moderate-intensity activities such as walking or household work—will increase the number of calories your body uses. The key to successful weight control and improved overall health is making physical activity a part of your daily routine.

What are the Health Benefits of Physical Activity?

In addition to helping to control your weight, research shows that regular physical activity can reduce your risk for several diseases and conditions and improve your overall quality of life. Regular physical activity can help protect you from the following health problems.

Heart Disease and Stroke

Daily physical activity can help prevent heart disease and stroke by strengthening your hart muscle, lowering your blood pressure, raising your high-density lipoprotein (HDL) levels (good cholesterol) and lowering low-density lipoprotein (LDL) levels (bad cholesterol), improving blood flow, and increasing your heart's working capacity.

High Blood Pressure

Regular physical activity can reduce blood pressure in those with high blood pressure levels. Physical activity also reduces body fatness, which is associated with high blood pressure.

Noninsulin-dependent Diabetes

By reducing body fatness, physical activity can help to prevent and control this type of diabetes.

Obesity

Physical activity helps to reduce body fat by building or preserving muscle mass and improving the body's ability to use calories. When physical activity is combined with proper nutrition, it can help control weight and prevent obesity, a major risk factor for many diseases.

Back Pain

By increasing muscle strength and endurance and improving flexibility and posture, regular exercise helps to prevent back pain.

Osteoporosis

Regular weight-bearing exercise promotes bone formation and may prevent many forms of bone loss associated with aging.

Studies on the psychological effects of exercise have found that regular physical activity can improve your mood and the way you feel about yourself. Researchers also have found that exercise is likely to reduce depression and anxiety and help you to better manage stress.

Keep these health benefits in mind when deciding whether or not to exercise. And remember, any amount of physical activity you do is better than none at all.

How Much Should You Exercise?

For the greatest overall health benefits, experts recommend that you do 20 to 30 minutes of aerobic activity three or more times a week and some type of muscle strengthening activity and stretching at least twice a week. However, if you are unable to do this level of activity, you can gain substantial health benefits by accumulating 30 minutes or more of moderate-intensity physical activity a day, at least five times a week.

If you have been inactive for a while, you may want to start with less strenuous activities such as walking or swimming at a comfortable pace. Beginning at a slow pace will allow you to become physically fit without straining your body. Once you are in better shape, you can gradually do more strenuous activity.

Moderate-intensity Activity

Moderate-intensity activities include some of the things you may already be doing during a day or week, such as gardening and housework. These activities can be done in short spurts—10 minutes here, 8 minutes there. Alone, each action does not have a great effect on your health, but regularly accumulating 30 minutes of activity over the course of the day can result in substantial health benefits.

To become more active throughout your day, take advantage of any chance to get up and move around. Here are some examples:

- Take a short walk around the block
- Rake leaves
- Play actively with the kids
- Walk up the stairs instead of taking the elevator
- Mow the lawn
- Take an activity break—get up and stretch or walk around
- Park your car a little farther away from your destination and walk the extra distance.

The point is not to make physical activity an unwelcome chore, but to make the most of the opportunities you have to be active.

Aerobic Activity

Aerobic activity is an important addition to moderate-intensity exercise. Aerobic exercise is any extended activity that makes you breathe hard while using the large muscle groups at a regular, even pace. Aerobic activities help make your heart stronger and more efficient. They also use more calories than other activities. Some examples of aerobic activities include:

- Brisk walking
- Jogging
- Bicycling
- Swimming

Aerobic dancing

Racket sports

Rowing

Ice or roller-skating

Cross-country or downhill skiing

Using aerobic equipment (*i.e.*, treadmill, stationary bike)

To get the most health benefits from aerobic activity, you should exercise at a level strenuous enough to raise your heart rate to your target zone. Your target heart rate zone is 50 to 75 per cent of your maximum heart rate (the fastest your heart can beat). To find your target zone, look for the category closest to your age in the chart below and read across the line. For example, if you are 35 years old, your target heart rate zone is 93-138 beats per minute.

Age Target	*Heart Rate*	*Zone 50-75%*	*Average Maximum Heart Rate 100%*
20-30 years	98-146 beats per min.	195	
31-40 years	93-138 beats per min.	185	
41-50 years	88-131 beats per min.	175	
51-60 years	83-123 beats per min.	165	
61+ years	78-116 beats per min.	155	

To see if you are exercising within your target heart rate zone, count the number of pulse beats at your wrist or neck for 15 seconds, then multiply by four to get the beats per minute. Your heart should be beating within your target heart rate zone. If your heart is beating faster than your target heart rate, you are exercising too hard and should slow down. If your heart is beating slower than your target heart rate, you should exercise a little harder.

When you begin your exercise programme, aim for the lower part of your target zone (50 per cent). As you get into better shape, slowly build up to the higher part of your target zone (75 per cent). If exercising within your target zone seems too hard, exercise at a pace that is comfortable for you. You will find that, with time, you will feel more comfortable exercising and can slowly increase to your target zone.

Stretching and muscle strengthening exercises; stretching and strengthening exercises such as weight training should also be a part of your physical activity programme. In addition to using calories, these exercises strengthen your muscles and bones and help prevent injury.

Tips to a Safe and Successful Physical Activity Programme

Make sure you are in good health. Answer the following questions before you begin exercising.

- Has a doctor ever said you have heart problems?
- Do you frequently suffer from chest pains?
- Do you often feel faint or have dizzy spells?
- Has a doctor ever said you have high blood pressure?
- Has a doctor ever told you that you have a bone or joint problem, such as arthritis, that has been or could be aggravated by exercise?
- Are you over the age of 65 and not accustomed to exercise?
- Are you taking prescription medications, such as those for high blood pressure?
- Is there a good medical reason, not mentioned here, why you should not exercise?

If you answered "yes" to any of these questions, you should see your doctor before you begin an exercise programme.

Follow a gradual approach to exercise to get the most benefits with the fewest risks. If you have not been exercising, start at a slow pace and as you become more fit, gradually increase the amount of time and the pace of your activity.

Choose activities that you enjoy and that fit your personality. For example, if you like team sports or group activities, choose things such as soccer or aerobics. If you prefer individual activities, choose things such as swimming or walking. Also, plan your activities for a time of day that suits your personality. If you are a morning person, exercise before you begin the rest of your day's activities. If you have more energy in the evening, plan activities that can be done at the end of the day. You will be more likely to stick to a physical activity programme if it is convenient and enjoyable.

Exercise Regularly

To gain the most health benefits it is important to exercise as regularly as possible. Make sure you choose activities that will fit into your schedule.

Exercise at a comfortable pace. For example, while jogging or walking briskly you should be able to hold a conversation. If you do not feel normal again within 10 minutes following exercise, you are exercising too hard. Also, if you have difficulty in breathing or feel faint or weak during or after exercise, you are exercising too hard.

Maximize your safety and comfort. Wear shoes that fit and clothes that move with you, and always exercise in a safe location. Many people walk in indoor shopping malls for exercise. Malls are climate controlled and offer protection from bad weather.

Vary your activities. Choose a variety of activities so you don't get bored with any one thing.

Encourage your family or friends to support you and join you in your activity. If you have children, it is best to build healthy habits when they are young. When parents are active, children are more likely to be active and stay active for the rest of their lives.

Challenge yourself. Set short-term as well as long-term goals and celebrate every success, no matter how small.

Whether your goal is to control your weight or just to feel healthier becoming physically active is a step in the right direction. Take advantage of the health benefits that regular exercise can offer and make physical activity a part of your lifestyle.

Natural Grooming Made Easy

The dictum 'beauty is skin deep' has to be reversed for our purpose of defining the good looks of your body as a whole. As, literally speaking, beauty is not skin deep—it's just the other way round. Your **looks** are the **mirror** of your body's and mind's internal condition. In other words, if you are healthy within, your skin and hair, your body and figure look beautiful too.

The skin is the biggest organ in our body which protects other internal organs and reflects the health of the body: placed close together, all over, the skin breathes, eliminates water, maintains the body temperature.

Minor skin eruptions find their way on most women's faces now and then even if she is basically healthy. The problem may start with adolescence when the sebacious (or oil producing glands) can become overproductive due to the hormonal changes prior to the early teens. Usually the face and neck are affected the most because of a larger number of oil glands in these areas. So keep in mind: whatever you do by way of treatment or care to the face skin, care should not stop at the chin but go right down to the base of your neck. An oily skin is prone to acne which can give way to pimples and infection and in turn these can leave their very long lasting marks. The pores get clogged with oil, causing white heads and when dust and make-up are not cleansed properly these turn to blackheads.

Before you decide on the preparation to apply during a daily care programme or you start any treatment at all, you should get to know about your skin type. Most skins can be of any one of the following four types: 1. Normal skin; 2. Oily skin; 3. Dry skin; 4. Would have combinations of oily and dry skins.

How do You Find Your Skin Type?

When you rise in the morning take a clean white tissue and wipe the centre of your cheeks and your forehead; have a good look at the tissue. If it's stained with oil, you have an oily skin, if not, that is, if the tissue continues to be dry and clean, wipe your nose and the area around it, and also your chin. If the result is an oily tissue this time then your skin is a combination of oily and dry, and needs (special double) care. However, if the tissue continues to be clean both times *i.e.,* even after wiping your nose and chin, you probably have a normal skin. Now to check if it's really normal and not dry, wash your face with soap and water. If the skin feels smooth and comfortable after you blot out the moisture you definitely have a normal skin. But on the contrary if it feels tight and stretched with the centre of the cheeks looking parched, soon after the wash, then you have a dry skin. But just make a mental note: Checking the skin on an excessively warm day when you perspire on the face may not give you the correct answer.

General foods should be cooked with as little oil and spice as possible. You can use all qualities of spices but don't use too much of them. Daily intake of curd and juice of half lemon in a little water taken every morning can also be very helpful. Lemon helps break down fat in the body and is rich in Vitamin 'C' which helps the skin get smoother.

If you are overweight or have a tendency towards it, neither lime nor curd should be sweetened. Only overly slim women and adolescents can use sugar. Papayas and pineapples are among the best fruits to help reduce weight and fresh watery fruits and vegetables like lettuce, cucumber, watermelons, etc., are very good for consumption as well as for external application on the facial skin. A slice of these fruits or their juice tone the skin when applied to the face. Raw carrots or their juice also help in the same way with Vitamin A.

Fresh mangoes and dry fruits are to be eaten sparingly because of their high-calorie content if you have a weight problem. Also, mangoes can precipitate skin eruptions. If you are underweight, and want to take lime juice daily because of an oily skin, it is suggested that you have at least a glass of pure milk daily and if you are non-veg, an egg on alternate days. However, if your weight is just normal, regular intake of skimmed milk will do. Always have fruits between meals, especially if you have digestion problems. If not, fruits can cause fermentation of food eaten at mealtime and consequently meals take longer to digest. Another important factor influencing skin quality is cleanliness.

Meticulous cleanliness is a must whatever your skin type. The number of times you wash with soap and water should depend upon how oily your skin is but routine cleansing at the end of your day should be compulsory.

Once you have discovered your skin type you can decide on the cosmetics to use according to our guidelines for a routine skin care. Whatever your skin type the soaps best suited for a wash are Ayurvedic soaps and glycerine soaps. The presently available ones are Chandrika Ayurvedic soap, Pears soap and glycerine soap. And again whatever your skin type a daily routine skin care session is a must for fresh and flawless skin.

This routine care will consist of four main processes: The first step is **cleansing** the skin of the day's perspiration, dust, grease and stale make-up. The next step would be **toning,** which will freshen up the skin and help get rid of any oil left over by cleansing creams or lotions. Skin tonics are usually astrigents and help tighten up the pores discouraging excess oil. Therefore, very mild astringents are advised for a dry skin.

The third step would be **moisturising** and this is imperative for all skin types. Dry skins need a generous splash of moisturizers. They can be used moderately on normal skins and sparingly on oily ones. And finally a **nourishing** cream or face mask can wind up your routine session.

Now let us deal in detail with the four operations with reference to each skin type:

A normal skin would be naturally smooth and easiest to care for. Wash once a day with soap and water, more times if you find it feeling a bit sticky. But removing dust and make-up in the evening needs a more efficient cleanser than plain soap and water. If you are reluctant to prepare your own cosmetics a good brand cleansing milk or cold cream would do. Milk and curd have oiling and softening properties so you can even use these which are definitely handy items in any household. You can give yourself a light massage or rather combine cleansing with a massage as you apply the cold cream and allow it to work on your skin before you wipe it off.

On the cheeks the cleanser should be spread with gentle yet inward circular firm strokes starting between the corners of the mouth and the nostrils going upwards below the eyes and stopping at the top of the ears. Alternate this circular motion of your fingers with one starting below the corners of the lips (*i.e.,* just above the corners of the mouth) but make a smaller semi-circle through the middle of your cheeks stopping at the ear holes.

After massaging the cheeks for a minute with these two strokes alternately you can deal with the jaw area: take some fresh cleanser on 3 middle finger tips of both your hands: Place the pointers just touching the lower sides of your nose and the other two fingers below the nose and move in horizontal strokes up to your ear lobes.

Massage this area for another minute. The eyes should be left out while dealing with the cheeks. The reason is the semi circle just below the eyelashes has very delicate skin which is usually more dry than the rest of the face and rough massaging can spoil the elasticity of the skin causing wrinkles earlier. If you use sour curd on the face, do not use it on the eyes. You can use a little milk. You could deal with the middle and index fingers, the eye area after you finish with the rest of the face. Start at the corners near the nose, each time, and go to the outer corners in semi-circular motion. Then starting and stopping at the same points as earlier, and using the same fingers, lightly massage the semi-circle below the eyes. Then place the fingers between the outer ends of the eyebrow and the corners of the eye.

Massage the moisturizer on the temples with a circular movement starting and ending on the same point and going up to the hairline. Next go up to the forehead; with four fingers of both hands used alternately, spread the moisturizer from the centre of the forehead to either side hairline. That is, the right hand going from middle of the forehead to right side hairline and then the left hand from middle of forehead to left side hairline; repeat with each hand till you feel the skin well massaged and stimulated. The cleanser would have been well absorbed by the forehead skin by now, and any dry make up loosened, but if you want to discourage wrinkles on this area, you could massage some more with the same finger tips.

Start at the middle of forehead and go to the right side hairline in small circles, then repeat with left hand from the middle to left side hair line. The direction of each circle should be away from the middle towards the respective side. You could repeat the operation starting lower down, starting between your eyebrows and moving your fingers high above the eyebrows to the temples and exerting a little pressure as you massage the temples in circular movements. This helps relaxation of nerve ends. Then massage the cleanser onto the chin also in circular movement with fingers of both hands. Pay attention to the jaw line or lower edge of your face; start at the tip of your chin and lightly drag the finger tips upto ear lobes. Don't leave out the neck; start at the middle base of your neck with the left hand and go just below the right ear, come back to the base and go to the middle section of the right side, and return to starting point and go over the lower section. Repeat twice. Then do same movements with right hand to spread the cleanser on the left side of the neck. And when you have done it, take care of the eyes, if you have left them out till now. The next step would be washing or cleaning off the cleanser along with the impurities that must be left loose on the skin.

The skin's worst enemy is the sun. If you avoid excessive sun exposure, you can help to prolong the youth and beauty of the skin. The sun can deprive the skin of moisture, hastening the appearance of those lines and wrinkles that ageing is all about. It is also responsible for many skin problems, like pigmentation, discolouration, freckles and even skin cancer. So, protect the skin with a sunscreen and moisturise it daily.

A moisturised cleanser that serves the dual purpose of cleansing and preventing moisture loss, would be ideal.

Dos and Don'ts

Water and detergents are the natural enemies of the skin for they cause dryness and even allergies. Always wear rubber gloves before dipping your hands in water, and massage with a rich, hand cream after every wash.

Petroleum jelly is a cheap and equally-effective substitute, if you don't like rubber gloves.

Apply liberally before putting your hands in water. Rub oil into your hands before cutting vegetables to prevent ugly stains.

Manicure and Pedicure

First remove oil nail enamel and file the nails. Massage hand cream into the nails and around the cuticles.

Soak hands and feet in warm, soapy water for 6 minutes. Scrub the feet with a pumice stone. Dry them and clean under the nails with cotton buds.

Massage a rich cream into the skin and wrap hands and feet in a towel wrung out in hot water. Dry well.

Apply nail polish in 3 coats, allowing each coat to dry before applying the next. Use smooth, straight strokes.

Common Complaints and their Cures

Rough hands and feet

Apply a paste of multani mitti, malai and honey on the hands for 20 minutes and wash off with cold water. Or, massage with a mixture of glycerine, almond oil and rose water.

Massage the feet with a mixture of a cup of salt and ¼ cup of water for 15 minutes. Rinse with warm water and apply a rich cream.

Cracked hands and feet

Use a zinc and castor oil ointment on the hands daily. For the feet, apply a mixture made of 2 tbsp hot coconut oil, ¼" piece of candle wax (melted) and 2 bits of camphor. Protect with a polythene wrapper for one hour.

Black marks and dark knuckles

Massage with a mixture of glycerine, lime juice and rose water, 15 minutes before a bath.

Brittle nails

Soak the nails in equal parts of hot coconut oil and hand lotion for 20 minutes, once a week. Or, soak daily in a cup of water to which a teaspoonful of gelatine has been added. Dry and massage with malai.

You can make your own multipurpose hand lotion by mixing $^{3}/_{4}$ cup of rose water, ¼ tsp white vinegar, ¼ cup of glycerine and ½ tsp honey.

For healthy hair, the right kind of food is very important. During the hot weather red meat and egg should be avoided completely as far as possible. Both these items generate body heat which in turn causes skin eruptions. A fresh-food, light diet is ideal—such as fish which is easily digestible, vegetables, fruits and salads. Plenty of liquids are a must-a minimum of 10 glasses of water plus 'chaas' and juices. As tempting as they are in the heat, fizzy drinks are very high in calories (80 calories per bottle).

Oily and fatty foods (junk food in particular) and also Chinese cuisine should be avoided in the heat. This high intake of oil merely serves to make the system feel sluggish. A good habit to acquire is that of soaking a handful of *channa* every night and eating them, freshly sprouted every morning on an empty stomach. Another beneficial tip is—have a glass of lukewarm water with a squeeze of lemon and a spoonful of honey on rising.

Hints on Hair Care

The Indian climate is often hot, humid and enervating: with it also arrive the problems of coping with hair that goes greasy in an hour, limp in a day and feels like a balaclava. Although one might yearn for a crew-cut in the heat or resort to desperate measures to deal with the grime, it is nevertheless important to remember that hair requires special care and attention during the summer months—and like any other part of the body, needs specific nutrients to maintain its health and quality. Here is all you need to know in order to cope with both your tresses and the heat—with elan.

A simple but effective basic routine can be as follows:

Massage and Conditioning

As far as possible oil-massage the hair and scalp before washing the hair. Although oil may seem the worst thing in summer, in fact it acts as a protective barrier to sun and water, and is the simplest and best conditioner. Heated oil is the simplest and best conditioner. Heated oil is the best as it is rapidly absorbed into the hair pores. Allow the oil to remain overnight (or at least 2-3 hours if the former is not possible) and wash off in the morning. The massage is very important.

The oil should be firmly (but not roughly) rubbed into the scalp, pressing pulse points to stimulate circulation, in rounded movements with the balls of the fingers. Never use nails to scratch the scalp. Specially remember to oil the hair tips to guard against split end. What oil to use? Coconut is a general favourite but almond, olive and castor oil are all beneficial. While once a week is an easy rule of thumb, in summer you may like to increase this routine to twice a week. For conditioning purpose, there are a variety of commercial products available, but in addition there are other conditioners which are often more effective and can be used once in two weeks. Of these, Amla is good for dry hair while henna benefits greasy hair. Henna will not colour black hair but will tinge grey hair. Egg is another source of protein. The white of an egg is used for greasy hair and the yolk for dry. The whole egg is used for normal hair. Another useful but not generally known tip is to use coconut milk in the hair, leave for two hours and then wash out. This leaves the hair shining and black.

Steaming

After a hot oil massage, steaming is excellent for circulation and opening of the pores. This can be done at a parlour or more easily (but equally effectively) at home merely by soaking a towel in hot, steaming water, wringing and then wrapping it turban-style round the head. Repeat the process every 10 minutes for half an hour. Once a week is sufficient.

Shampooing

Most people do not give this process a second thought—but please do, as it has a lasting effect on your hair. Rinse hair thoroughly. Do not bunch up hair but allow the water to run from the nape to head-top and down to tips. Running water is best used for this. Pour shampoo onto palm: not directly onto the hair as this means it soaks into one spot instead of spreading evenly. Massage scalp in the same way as with oil (round and round with finger tips) and down to the very tips. Do not treat tips roughly. Wash out thoroughly, again without bunching and screwing the hair. Shampoo residue causes flaking on the scalp which is often mistaken for dandruff. For those with greasy hair, shampoo a second time leaving it for five minutes before rinsing. Hair should feel squeaky clean when finished.

Many people prefer not to use shampoos. Good substitutes are shikakai soap or reetha. How often should one wash hair in summer? The safest and best guide is—when you feel your hair is dirty-be it every day, every second day or every few days—but never less than once a week. Frequent washing does not damage hair if it is conditioned properly. Treat hair like any other part of your body—when dirty or sweaty, wash it-but in the way described. Shampoos facilitate easy washing, quick drying and combing. Liquid shampoos are most popular. These are made of sodium or potassium salts, lauryl sulphates, solubilising agents, foam stabilisers, preservatives, emmolients, thickening agents, etc.

Special ingredients like lemon, herbs, lanolin, egg, antiseptics and anti-dandruff agents, are also sometimes added.

One should not go by the quantity of lather formation, as the cleansing property of a shampoo has nothing to do with it. One should be careful in the choice of a shampoo to avoid irritation to the eyes, scalp and neck, and the thinning of hair.

A brisk morning walk is excellent as the ozone in the atmosphere is good for the system. Running, jogging, cycling, etc.—are all a matter of preference. Whatever the means, do not forget to set aside 10 minutes minimum for daily regimen. For the lazy, bathroom exercises are the easiest solution (do not cheat on the toe-touching). Another excellent idea is yoga (10-15 minutes a day is not much to ask). Apart from benefitting the body, its meditative principle relieves mental tensions and leaves you better able to cope with your day and its problems.

(a) **Greasy Hair:** Follow the basic routine of massage and shampooing suggested earlier. Contrary to popular belief, one should not omit the oil massage, but do wash out thoroughly with two rinses. In the last rinse add juice of half lemon to the water. Do not hesitate to wash daily if necessary as greasy hair attracts pollutants to the scalp.

(b) **Dry Hair:** Dry hair tends to become brittle in the heat. Oil thoroughly—castor oil has a heavy base and is very good for this problem. Also use a daily cream every morning. Amla is a good conditioning agent.

(c) **Dandruff:** Most lay people are unaware that dandruff can be of two types—dry and greasy. The former is usually noticeable as it is flaky and falls. The latter, however, often goes undetected as it sticks to the greasy scalp and does not detach easily. However, it is equally bad for the hair which often falls as a consequence. Contrary to popular belief, dandruff is not dead cells but in fact a living organism—a parasite. The main causes of dandruff are poor circulation, lack of nerve stimulation, improper diet, emotional disturbance, lack of hygiene and dryness. It is also highly infectious and can be passed on through combs or other contact. Thus it becomes very important to keep combs and towels separate, even within the family or between siblings. Another common problem due to dandruff is pimples, acne or a rash on the face and shoulders.

How to Tackle Dandruff: There is no quick remedy. The normally suggested line of treatment by beauty parlours is the use of medicated shampoos such as Selsun or Clinic. Over a period of time they succeed in substantially reducing, if not curing altogether, the problem.

(d) **Falling Hair:** There are cases of balding or sudden hair loss which require proper diagnosis by a beauty dermatologist. It is however, normal to lose 60-75 hairs a day. Hair is often affected by emotional disturbances, physical causes, tension or environmental factors such as water and air. A good routine to follow is a hot oil massage, followed by steam and a mild shampoo. Diet should include sprouted *channa* every morning and if the cause is physical weakness—iron capsules. For the relief of tension Kali Phos 6 X (a bio-chemic remedy) is both harmless and effective. For severe hair loss do not waste any time in consulting a beauty-dermatologist.

(e) **Lice:** Another nuisance, but one which must be treated every day. Apply strong lye soap or shampoo after combing (with a fine comb) dipped in Dettol solution. Wash combs and brushes scrupulously in lye solution.

Cosmetics

The term 'cosmetics' includes a wide range of products intended for application to any part of our body—for cleaning, beautifying and enhancing our appearance.

These include dentifrices, toilet soaps, face powders, creams, hair preparations, nail preparations and other make-up aids, like lipstick, rouge, mascara, etc. Such products abound in the market.

Let us briefly survey these various preparations.

Dentifrices: Popular dentifrices used with a toothbrush include toothpaste and powder.

A wide range of commercial preparations, each claiming to have a unique formula to prevent tooth decay, gum trouble and bad breath, is available in the market.

Most consumers are guided by flavours in selecting a toothpaste. Some keep changing brands and get carried away by advertisements, little knowing that all pastes have the same ingredients in them, except for different flavouring oils. A toothpaste is made up of the following ingredients.

Common Ingredients

1. A mild abrasive agent, like calcium carbonate, hydrated alumina, etc.
2. A small quantity of synthetic detergent, like sodium lauryl sulphate to penetrate the narrow spaces between the teeth and to facilitate the removal of foreign matter during rinsing.
3. A humectant like glycerol, sorbitol, to keep the paste from drying out (A humectant is a moisturing agent).
4. Binders to prevent the separation of the liquid ingredients from the solid ones during storage. A natural gum from karaya, seaweed, or cellulose derivatives are used for this purpose.
5. **Flavours and Sweeteners:** Each brand of paste has its own flavour, like peppermint, aniseed, cinnamon, clove, eucalyptus, etc. These are blended with sweeteners, like saccharin, to make it palatable.

6. Special ingredients, like fluoride, chlorophyll, etc. which are advertised as being beneficial for the teeth.

   While fluoride is known to help teeth to become resistent to tooth decay, dentists are still divided in their opinion on the merits of incorporating fluoride in tooth pastes, for an excess of fluoride can cause mottling of teeth and other disorders.

   Peroxides and antibacterials, like hexachlorophene and penicilin, which have disinfectant properties were once thought to be desirable for oral use. However, it is no longer considered so, as they are known to destroy the natural flora of the mouth and to cause injury to the mucous membrane of the mouth.

   This unnatural interference with the microbial equilibrium in the mouth can have adverse long ranging effects. Hence, they are not necessary for normal dental hygiene.

   No particular toothpaste can afford total protection against dental decay. Any ordinary toothpaste with a good cleaning action, oral hygience and good dietary habits, can do more for the teeth than a total reliance on the exaggerated claims of 'unique' toothpastes.

Talcum Powders

The largest selling of all cosmetics, talcum powder is used as a finishing touch to the make-up process. Face powders serve to cover up minor blemishes on the skin and impart a smooth finish to the face bringing about a certain shine.

Hydrated magnesium silicate is the most important component of powders. Good and fine quality talc makes the powder soft and fluffy and helps it to spread evenly over the face. To help it adhere to the skin, magnesium stearates are used.

To improve absorbency, calcium carbonate or kaolin is used. Colour-pigments and perfumes enhance its appeal.

In selecting a powder, one must see if the powder spreads evenly and is capable of absorbing perspiration. A good powder should blend well, look natural and be delicately perfumed. Talcs with bactericides should not be used, especially for babies, and on the face.

Face Creams

Cold creams, cleansing creams and vanishing creams have flooded the market. Cold creams and cleansing creams are emulsions of mineral oil, like bee wax, parafiin oil, borax and water. In addition, they contain perfumes, emmolients preservatives and floral waters.

These have good cleansing properties because of their solvent action. They can help remove make-up and grime from the skin in a better way than soap.

But they also dissolve out the skin fat and hence there is a need to lubricate treated skin. Cold cream, made from vegetable oil, can help protect the skin against drying, and would also nourish the skin.

Creams made from mineral oils, cannot nourish the skin as mineral oil is not absorbed by the skin.

Paraffin and lanolin are also added along with the perfumes to make the cream richer, light and fluffy.

Vanishing creams contain stearic acid, alkali, water and a humectant like glycerine. Vanishing cream leaves a pearly film on the skin. It is prized for its ability to retain a thin film of make-up for a long period. However, in case of excessive use it can cause a dry burning sensation. A good cream must give a good matt finish and be stable under various climatic conditions.

Hand Lotions and Creams

These are made with glycerine, rosewater, boric acid and perfumed oils. They help in preventing roughness and chapping of hands and help to keep the skin supple and smooth for those engaged in manual cleaning and washing.

Nail Polish

Nail enamel is made up of the following ingredients:

A film-forming substance like nitro-celluloe, plasticizers to provide plasticity, a solvent to control its viscosity and colourants, using inorganic pigments for the desired shades.

The 'frosted' lacquers contain transparent pearl-like crystals of mica flakes or fish scale extracts.

A good nail lacquer should adhere to the nail and be resistant to chipping and abrasion. It should not stain the nail or irritate the skin, and should be fast in colour. For sensitive people, nail lacquers could cause skin lesions.

Lipsticks

Looking like bright crayons, lipsticks come in a wide range of shades—brilliant plains and frosted hues. Common ingredients in lipsticks are waxes, oils, fats to provide lubrication, perfumes, and colourants, preservatives and anti-oxidants to prevent rancidity.

Lipsticks are used for beauty and to prevent lips from cracking in cold weather. Hence, they should be chosen with care as they could be absorbed into the body and prove toxic, if inferior in quality.

A good lipstick should be nontoxic and retain its consistency even during prolonged storage. It should give a smooth appearance to the lips without sweating, drying out or cracking. It should be water resistant.

Its indiscreet use may result in red scaling, fissures, crusts and swelling of lips because of the presence of certain harmful colourants or dyes.

Eye Make-up

Lamp-black or carbon black is widely used as urma or *kajal* for darkening or beautifying eyes. Mascara is a vaseline preparation, containing a black dye.

Lead poisoning, impairment of vision or loss of eyesight may result through its indiscreet use.

Hair Dyes

These are used to conceal grey hair. In these vegetable colouring, metal salts and oxidation dyes are used. 'Shampoo-in' dyes and cream formulations are both popular, but one must take a preliminary test to rule out allergic reactions.

Frequent dyeing can cause hair damage and sensitisation of scalp, neck, ears, or cause weeping eczema.

Unwanted Hair

Unwanted hair is removed by using depilatories which detach hair at the skin level. They come in powder, paste, cream or liquid forms.

Before their application to larger areas, one should test them for allergy, which may cause pain or trauma because of the presence of thioglycolates or sulphides. A lot of synthetic chemicals go into the preparation of modern cosmetics. We may make the mistake of using them without properly being aware of the potential health hazards, particularly for children.

Many cosmetics especially low-quality products, can cause irritation, dermatitis, blockage of sweat glands, headache, asthma, respiratory allergy, blood disorders, discomfort or damage to eyes and even cancer.

Perfumes

Did you know that perfumes were classified in groups on the basis of one or more identifiable dominant odours? They are:

1. **Floral:** These blend odours such as jasmine, rose, lily of the valley and gardenia.
2. **Spicy:** These blends feature such aromas as carnation, clove, cinnamon and nutmeg.
3. **Woody:** This group is characterised by such odours as vetiver (or khuskhus), sandalwood and cedarwood.
4. **Mossy:** This family is dominated by oak moss.
5. **Orientals:** This collection combines woody, mossy and spicy notes with such sweet odours as vanilla or balsam, and is usually accentuated by animal odours.
6. **Animal:** These include musk or civet.
7. **Herbal:** These are characterised by clover and sweet grass odours.
8. **Leather and tobacco:** they feature aromas of leather, tobacco and smokiness of birchtar.
9. **Aldehydic group:** These are dominated by odours of the aromatic chemicals (aldehydes), usually having a fruity character.

Fine perfumes contain more than a 100 ingredients. Each perfume is composed of a top note, the refreshing, volatile odour perceived immediately, a middle note, or modifier, providing full, solid character, and a base note also called an end note or basic note which is most persistent.

Then again, perfume concentrates are in different proportions for:

1. Perfumes or handkerchief perfumes—10-25%.
2. Toilet water and cologne—2-6%.
3. After-shave lotions and splash colognes—2-6%.

The next part is for those who are all for ingenuity and love experimenting with novel ideas. Here then, are listed some hints to ensure a perfumed aura around them.

1. Spray cologne on damp, towel-dried hair before combing—how delightfully charming!
2. Dab a few drops of perfume on light bulbs and tubelights—when switched on, the heat will diffuse fragrance. How's that for novelty?
3. Tuck scent-saturated cotton balls in pillow cases—sweet dreams, folks!
4. Spray cologne on the underside of wooden bookshelves, the scent will linger on for ages—bookworms needn't sneeze amidst gammexane anymore!
5. Store scented soap, unwrapped, in lingerie. You've got a wide choice in scents this way.
6. Dab cologne on a sheet of plain bond paper, let dry and keep it under business papers in your briefcase. Hmmm, business and pleasure, is it?
7. Pick up rug and carpet corners and spray the undersides with cologne.
8. Scented hankies can be tucked into the corner of your purse the lacier the prettier!
9. Store all your empty perfume bottles in bureau drawers, till all traces of fragrance vanish—for maximum 'consumer satisfaction.'
10. Spray perfume on the khus in your cooler—sit back to be pleasantly surprised at the fragrant results.

11. Put perfume on the petal of artificial flowers.
12. Spray fabric-covered hangers in the clothes closet—now, isn't that ingenious!
13. Spray perfume on your bra before putting it on in the morning.

Beauty Aids from Your Kitchen

Lemon, the pale yellow citrus fruit, which is an almost indispensable item in our regular marketing list can be an important beauty aid.

To purchase juicy lemons, it is best to go in for the big, round, ripe yellow ones with thin rinds. If they get hard due to storage they can be soaked in hot water for sometime, before being squeezed.

A healthy lemon contains 4 to 5% of citric acid. It is a veritable storehouse of beauty remedies.

It can be used as a natural beauty conditioner. Cut a lemon into half and squeeze out the juice. Add some plain water and a few drops of rosewater.

Apply with cotton wool on the face and keep for sometime before washing off. It leaves the skin soft and petal-smooth.

For very oily skins, the white of an egg can be added to the juice of half a lemon. After keeping it on for 10 minutes, the face can be washed with tepid water and soap.

The best and easiest home remedy for rough, broken skin is given below.

To one teaspoonful of gramflour, a spoonful of fresh milk or milk cream is to be added. A pinch of turmeric and the juice of a quarter piece of a lemon should be mixed with this to form a smooth paste. This paste is to be applied to the face and neck. Remove after lightly massaging with the hands. Wash the face and neck with lukewarm water.

This method, followed once a week, or even a fortnight, works wonders on the complexion.

Lemon juice mixed with honey is an effective remedy for removing dark spots on the body. Plain lemon, cut into two halves, can be 'cupped' into the elbows for a short time regularly, to make the elbows palpably soft and to develop a lighter tinge.

After squeezing a lemon, just brush the skin over your hands, nails or neck before disposing it off. This will act as a natural astringent.

Lemon and hair share a perfect rapport. Directly pouring water on the hair is not the appropriate manner of a healthy hairwash. In case you have misgivings about the use of an egg, well, just squeeze the juice of a lime on your scalp and massage gently.

After 10 or 15 minutes, wash with either shikakai, gramflour or shampoo. This helps not only in getting rid of (and the prevention of) dandruff, but also bestows a healthy lustre to the hair.

Squeezing a couple of drops of lemon juice into the water, while bathing, makes us feel refreshed.

In the wide-ranging search for the secrets of beauty, women have turned time and again to the kitchen, the rationale being that if foods are good for you when taken into the body, then they must be beneficial when they are used on the outside of the body. Cucumber, eggs, vinegar, oatmeal, papaya—the list goes on and on. But at the forefront of the long line of edible cosmetics is the golden honey.

Honey has long been recognised as a perfect, all-round rejuvenator. It is mentioned in the Bible and the Koran. The ancients valued it not only as a food but as a medicine for internal and external use. It was considered invaluable as a remedy for burns and lacerations.

But the uses to which honey has been put over the years seem unlimited. The thick liquid soothes, heals and nourishes. Spread on the skin, it produces baby-soft smoothness even though only a fraction is actually absorbed by the skin. The many vitamins and minerals in honey make it a potent combatant of undernourished skin with its clogged and muddy look. Repeated applications of tissue-building honey will bring a glow of colour where none existed before. Honey is believed to contain antiseptic qualities. Applied to inflamed skin, it will kill bacteria and restore health.

Honey as Face Mask

Moreover, this delicious food for the bees is easy to use. For more youthful appearance the following simple facial produces impressive results. Splash warm water across a freshly washed face. Do not use any other preparation other than an astringent lotion after cleaning. Other cosmetics will create a film barrier over the very pores you are trying to reach. Reserve your creams for later.

Dip two fingers into a teaspoonful of honey (raw honey is preferred). In upward sweeping motions, lightly spread it over every area of your face. Be sure your hair is drawn back and your face fully exposed to the ear lobes and the top of the forehead for this facial honey bath.

Allow the honey to remain on your face for twenty minutes. Then rinse away with warm water. Daily applications of honey can refine and soften skin that has hardened from exposure and poor care. Honey is also helpful to use after removing make-up. Directly after its use a final rinse in a mixed solution of apple cider, vinegar and water will bring a further glow to the skin.

The glory of using one's kitchen as a beauty workshop is that many of the ingredients are already there. As long as you keep a jar of honey on your shelf, half the battle against early wrinkles is won. One quickie treatment that can soften the early wrinkling areas around the eyes, mouth and forehead consists of combining one teaspoonful of honey with two tablespoonfuls of cream. Be sure the cream is not 'milk food' or other substitutes.

Honey & Cream

Beat the honey and cream together and apply to a freshly scrubbed, rinsed and dried face. With the fingertips, pat the mixture into creases and lines. With a gentle rubbing action, saturate the grooved lines. Spread the lines on your face apart as you apply the honey and cream. Don't pull or work roughly. Smooth the area instead and attempt to increase the lines.

Another kitchen treatment using honey requires an equally minimal amount of preparation. Mix one-half teaspoonful of apple cider, vinegar or lime juice with two tablespoonfuls of honey. Blend together and spread over the face. Allow this to remain on for twenty minutes before rinsing away in warm water and blotting the skin dry. This softens and deep cleans leaving the skin refreshed and free of accumulated oils that a cleansing cream cannot reach. And don't forget the neck.

Honey & Almonds

One of the finest cosmetic teams available is honey and almonds in combination. The qualities of both have long been recognised by women the world over who have mastered the art of looking their best at all times. This old recipe, in all its grand simplicity, is really like having a pot of gold on hand. It's a truly effective skin preserver and a rejuvenator.

Buy a half-pound jar of U.S.P. lanolin (U.S.P. means it is approved for pharmaceutical use). Place one-fourth of a pound of good quality honey in the top of a double boiler. As it warms, beat in the half-pound of lanolin. As this melts, add one half cup of sweet almond oil and stir until well blended.

Remove from the heat and beat thoroughly with an electric beater. Let it thicken and then pour into convenient-sized jars. Keep all but the jar you are using in the refrigerator. Label the jars carefully so they aren't mistaken for food. Use the cream liberally over neck, face and elbows. And watch the magic it creates when you step out smelling of honey and almond cream.

Honey comes to the rescue again for victims of the sun. It chases away those awful red and brown blotches sometimes caused by India's scorching orb. When mixed with oatmeal it will soften and clear the skin as the oatmeal acts as a mild bleach. If used by night and rinsed away each morning, the following mixture will give a sparkling appearance.

Honey Paste

Mix the following items together until you have an easily spreadable paste: one ounce of honey, one teaspoonful of lime juice, two unbeaten egg whites, one-half-teaspoonful sweet almond oil and enough oatmeal powder to make a smooth paste. (Try whirling a handful of plain old-fashioned oatmeal in the mixer/blender for this, or use a mortar and pestle). The mixture should be moist but not dripping when you apply it.

When used sensibly and with dedication in these suggested mixtures, honey should go far to ward off the unwelcome aspects of age brought on by neglect of the body.

Cosmetics and How to Use them

Every woman has on hand the cosmetics she uses frequently. Lipstick, eyeliner, may be a bindi—that's what most of us own. But to present a completely made-up face that accentuates your attractive features, and generally gives you that polished look, it is a must to keep a complete range of cosmetics.

Start off with a toner to clean your skin. Depending on your skin type, you should use either an astringent (for oily skin) or a skin tonic (if your skin is normal to dry). A toner removes oil from your face; an oily face does not retain make-up for long.

Moisturizer

Next is a moisturiser to keep your skin soft and retain your skin's natural moisture. This is especially important as you grow older, and your skin loses its elasticity.

Anyone who uses make-up must use some kind of base, either a foundation or moisturiser, on her skin. This protects your face against the effects of ageing, and of pollution—so abrasive in our cities—as well as any harsh chemicals in the make-up. An additional use of foundation is to cover any small blemishes and irregularities. If you want to disguise a flaw, use a darker shade of foundation in that area; if you want to highlight a feature, use a lighter shade. You can use either a liquid make-up—choose a shade which most closely matches your skin colour—or the pancake variety, which is less popular, and used more for stage artistes. Some women don't like the artificial feeling of foundation, in which case they use a moisturiser as a base. Foundations are available in several shades.

Removing Make-up

After a wild night out partying with your prettily made-up face, don't forget to take it off when you come home. A cleansing lotion will remove all traces of make-up—in fact, you should use it before you put anything on your face. And again, use a toner to take off all traces of oil before you drop off to sleep.

Use cold cream and clean it up with a tissue. After you have wiped the complete make-up rinse your face in cold water, towel dry and use alcohol-free lotion toner on cotton cosmetic pad for final cleaning. For oily skin use an alcohol-based astringent for cleaning. Remove eye make-up with baby oil.

How to remove lipstick?

Squirt some baby oil into a paper tissue and wipe your lips.

Most of the sophisticated cosmetics available today are based on the good old concoctions. Any why not, those old beauty aids really worked! So perhaps it's time to rediscover some of those magic remedies which are designed to bring out the best in a women...

Your make-up kit must have all those extras-nail polish remover, cuticle softener, cotton balls, the different brushes for applying the make-up, etc. And buy a good air brush that won't pull your hair or scratch your scalp. Hairspray is useful to keep an elaborate hairstyle in place, but it must be used sparingly. Your purse should contain a 'repair box' powder compact, lipstick, comb, etc. to keep you going through a long evening.

When you apply mascara, moisten it with a skin freshner instead of water. This will help to eliminate the dry effect.

To make sparse eyelashes appear thicker, apply mascara, wait till it is dry, then pat face powder on the lashes. Then apply another coat. This will make them appear longer and luxuriant.

Dark circles are caused by eye strain or lack of vitamins. Dark circles are also hereditary. Get yourself checked by a doctor to rule out any organic problem. Whitening cream will not help. You can massage the area under the eyes with any good enriched cream.

Scanty Eyebrows

Make sure that the eye pencil is pointed and grease-free. When touching up your eyebrows use light, feathery strokes. This will prevent an unnatural hard line.

Dry Lips

Massage your lips with a little glycerine dissolved in water. Malai (milk cream) is also good. Apply a moisturiser at a night to keep your lips soft and smooth.

Scanty Hair

To combat dry hair, oil it regularly with olive oil. If you have dandruff, use medicated shampoo. Avoid using hand dryers. For a fuller effect, you can set your hair in rollers.

Hair Eye for Grey Hair

There are temporary colours, semi-permanent rinses and tints. Temporary colours are those which add a transparent coating of colour to the hair, but do not penetrate the hair shaft.

Semi-permanent rinses last for four or five shampoos and penetrate the hair shaft to some extent. There are a safe step between temporary rinses and more durable colours. Tints penetrate the hair shaft and cannot be shampooed out immediately. They last for a couple of months. But the roots have to be touched up as the hair grows.

Straight Hair

These days perms do not necessarily means curls. What your hair needs is a body wave perm which will give it a volume and lift, without curling it. Body wave works particularly well on slightly layered hair, but does not look so good on very long hair of even length. First have a good hair cut and then a body wave.

How often to use Henna

You can henna your hair once a month for a good shine. If you have a few strands of grey hair, then you have to do it once in three weeks.

Henna is known to have been used for colouring the hair and as a conditioner.

Take two cups of henna powder, 2 eggs, 1½ cup curds, 2 tsps instant coffee powder, (for oily hair add decoction of 2 tsps tea leaves). Mix and keep overnight. Apply to each strand of hair. Wash off after 45 minutes if used as a conditioner and after three hours if used for colour. Amla or lime juice added to the mixture and kept in an iron vessel, will give the hair a black tint.

Hibiscus leaves ground to a paste and applied to the hair acts as a conditioner and gives your hair a shiny look.

Dandruff

Dandruff can be got rid off when simple and inexpensive methods. Make a paste of multani mitti (fullers earth) and water. Apply it to the scalp and wash off after five minutes. Do not allow to dry.

A mixture of one egg, half cup curd (juice of one lime for oily hair) applied to the scalp and washed off after half an hour has been found to be an effective remedy for dandruff.

Another effective home remedy for dandruff is a mixture of one tsp fenugreek (methi) powder added to one egg and applied to the scalp for 10 minutes.

Greying Hair

Greying hair is not considered a major problem any more. A simple home-made treatment with 'trifla' water can check it in its initial stages itself. Take *amla, harde* and *behede,* in equal quantity. Soak in water in an iron vessel. Strain the water and apply at the roots of the hair. This is for hair in the initial stages of greying.

Falling Hair

For thick growth of hair and to check premature greying, a mixture of coconut oil and mustard oil should be heated with trifla water until all the water evaporates and only the oil remains. This oil can be stored and applied daily.

Another easy solution for falling hair is a mixture of coconut milk and goat's milk applied to the scalp.

Attractive Eye Lashes

For sparse eyelashes apply castor oil on the eyelids and lashes every night before sleeping. For sparkling eyes try washing them in an eyeglass with *trifla* water. Tired eyes can be given the same treatment with rose water instead, or even teabags or cucumber slices.

Dark Circles

Nobody wants dark circles under the eyes. Here's an effective remedy for it. Grind to a paste two almonds soaked in one tbsp of milk. Add four drops of lime juice and two drops of honey. Apply around the eyes. Wash off after an hour.

Face...

Today the 'in thing' is to have a facial regularly. It is supposed to tighten sagging skin as well as get rid of dull and dead skin. Beauticians use a whole lot of creams for the facial massage. But the age-old remedy of 'malai' (fresh cream) is probably still the most effective. For a glowing complexion try massaging your face with this: Mix one fourth tsp haldi with one tbsp malai and a few drops of lime juice. Rub this on your face and remember that the strokes must always be in an upward and outward direction. Oily skin can be massaged with dahi (curd).

Freckles & Black Heads

Say goodbye to unwanted freckles by applying juice of red mulli (radish).

Warts can be got rid off with cauliflower juice.

If black-heads is your major problem, you can try fomenting them with a solution of half cup boiling water and half tsp baking soda. The blackheads get loosened and you can easily press them out.

Fair Complexion

To lighten their complexion, many women use whitening creams or bleach their faces regularly. But, the use of ammonia can cause a lot of damage to an otherwise good skin. A few home remedies to lighten the colour of the skin are more advisable. Soak four almonds overnight. Peel the skin and grind to a fine paste. Mix in one tsp of gram flour, one tsp fresh, unboiled milk and a few drops of lime juice. Make a thick paste and apply on the face and neck. Leave it on for 15 minutes then massage gently into the skin until it comes off. Rinse face with cold water.

Massaging the face each morning with coconut water too is supposed to help lighten the complexion.

Acne and Pimples

It is caused due to hormonal imbalances and sometimes even if one is constipated. First go to a dermatologist, get yourself checked and simultaneously get it also treated by a therapist. The best way for such skin is wash twice daily with a soap or cleaner that is specially formulated for oily skin. Never squeeze your pimples because this will cause infection and even erupt more. There are also special cover-up cakes and creams in the markets.

How often should one go for facials?

Between 20 to 30 years, once a month, 20 to 40 twice a month and above 40 once a week.

Dark Patches

Dark patches on the skin can be got rid off by rubbing them with the juice of the leaves of ridge gourd (turai).

An excellent whitening lotion is one tbsp of cucumber juice, a few drops of lime juice and a dash of turmeric powder applied over the face for fifteen minutes every day.

Age-old Home Cosmetics

From time immemorial Indian women have made cosmetics out of material easily found in the market and used in their kitchen. These natural items have proved themselves as effective cosmetics or as principal ingredients in their making. We start with a list of readily available food products which have been traditionally used as natural cosmetics.

Almond — should be crushed to make masks, good for nourishing the skin.

Alum — has astringent properties and can be used in lotions.

Banana — can be used as a mask for dry skin.

Barley — rich in vitamin B and iron. Excellent tonic for overall nourishment and cleansing.

Buttermilk — is used as a cleanser. It also has bleaching properties and can be used for pigmentation.

Cabbage — rich in vitamins and minerals. Wash face with the water it has been cooked in.

Castor oil — rich oil used to thicken hair growth.

Corn milk — is a good pack for dry skins.

Cucumber — has slight astringent properties and is excellent for oily skins.

Eggs — The most useful aid to beauty. The yolk is nourishing and the white has tightening properties. It is used in mask and in hair conditioners.

Fullers Earth (Multani matti) — absorbent clay. It is rich in minerals, used as masks, has stimulating qualities.

Gelatine — has proteins-a good nail hardener.

Henna (Mehndi) — is a natural dye and an excellent conditioner for hair.

Honey — it has softening qualities. It is nourishing and used in masks and creams.

Iodine — white iodine is excellent for fungus infected nails.

Lettuce — rich in vitamins, iron and minerals. It is cooling and excellent for sunburns.

Mint — is a good natural cure for scars, pimple marks and skin disorders.

Oatmeal — is an excellent cleanser, often used in masks.

Onions — its juice prevents blemishes and mixed with honey makes a wonderful anti-wrinkle cream.

Papaya — breaks down the dead cells of skin and cleanses it. It is used as masks.

Potatoes — use thin slices as eye pads to remove puffiness under the eyes.

Salt — mixed with equal amount of soda bicarbonate makes an excellent cleanser for the teeth.

Sesame Oil — absorbs ultraviolet rays and is used for tanning the skin.

Strawberry — is excellent for discolouration. Stained teeth can be cleaned with its juice.

Tea — is a soother and is good to relax eyes. Keep cold tea pads on the eyes for severe dark circles.

Tomato — contains vitamin C. It is used to cleanse blackheads and close open pores.

Vinegar — is an excellent conditioner. Mixed with equal parts of water rinse hair after shampooing.

Yogurt — has cleansing properties and is used in face masks.

Controlling Pimples & Acne

These age-old methods of controlling pimples and acne are, in our view, the most effective of all methods.

1. Steam the face in water to which crushed neem leaves have been added. This is an effective way of controlling pimples.
2. Boil neem leaves in a little water. Strain, add the water to Multani Mitti (Fuller's earth) and make a paste. This pack will discourage pimples.
3. Make a paste of Kasturi haldi (turmeric) and apply it on the face and neck. This pack not only helps in controlling pimples, but also gives the skin a healthy glow.
4. Mint leaves are effective in treating pimples. The juice extracted from mint leaves should be applied on the face before going to bed. This treatment should be followed for a month.
5. Make a paste of equal amounts of sandalwood and turmeric. Apply to the face and neck and wash off after an hour. Sandalwood, by itself, is also effective in treating pimples.
6. Camphor is a good astringent. Apply camphor lotion to the affected areas before going to bed and wash off in the morning with a mild medicated soap and lukewarm water.
7. Dry orange peels thoroughly and powder them in a mixer. Mix the powder required for the time with a little milk and apply it to the affected areas. Wash off after an hour.

Cleaning Blackheads

Honey and milk are two effective mediums of clearing the face of blackheads.

Warm a little honey and apply it on the face. Wash off after 20 minutes. Or wash the face with warm water and sponge with lukewarm milk for 20 minutes.

Precautions:

1. Wash face with warm water and medicated soap frequently. Lather the soap into the pores thoroughly. Do not rub hard with towel. Dry gently.
2. After washing, a drying lotion or cream may be used. Alcohol, which is a drying lotion, may be used for the purpose.
3. Take plenty of fresh fruits and vegetables.
4. Fried foods and sweets should be avoided.

5. Tie your hair back or keep it short. Hair falling on the face can increase the pimples. If you have dandruff, get it treated, for the scales dropping on the face and neck can cause acne.
6. Never squeeze or pick at the pimples and acne spots. This will lead to the infection spreading to other parts.
7. Don't use greasy cosmetics. Choose cosmetics with a non-greasy base. Avoid using foundations since they tend to increase the blemishes on the skin.

Here are some preparations:

- Mix together a little sandalwood powder, camphor lotion, lime juice and multani mitti. Apply over the affected areas and allow to dry. Wash off with cold water.
- Paste of *pudina* leaves (mint leaves) has been known to dry up pimples or any other skin rash.
- An old but effective treatment for pimples is a thick paste of starch applied over the affected areas.
- Another effective remedy is a paste of gram flour, turmeric powder, crushed neem leaves and milk.
- A paste of multani mitti and water helps tighten pores that may be left open after an attack of pimples.
- To remove dead skin apply a mixture of glycerine, lime juice and sugar rubbing it into the skin gently.
- If your skin lacks lustre, try massaging it with a mixture of an equal amount of baby oil and table salt.
- Mash a ripe banana and mix in a little rose water. Apply it thickly over the face. Wash off with warm water after an hour. This not only keeps pimples at bay but also softens the skin and keeps it wrinkle-free.
- Add a little carrot juice to a cup of milk and rub this into the face if suffering from chicken pox marks or blemishes.
- To remove wrinkles and laugh lines apply a mixture of a tbsp of honey and one-fourth tsp of carrot juice. Leave it on for 15 minutes. Wash off with warm water.
- To remove pimple marks and blemishes make coarse rice powder. Mix in honey, lime juice and curd. Make a thick

paste and apply it over the face. Leave it on till half dry. Then rub off gently in circular movements.

Face Packs

Home-made face packs are rich in proteins—just what an under-nourished skin craves for. Egg is probably one of the best suppliers of proteins and can be used as a base for any kind of face pack. The only thing to be remembered is that the yolk is good only for dry skin while the white is excellent for an oily one. Here are some easy-to-make face-packs which have to be used to be believed. The effect can be phenomenal.

Soak one cup rice in water overnight. Strain and dry. Powder it with one inch piece of multani mitti and a teasponful of methi (fenugreek seeds). Store this in a jar. This powder should be mixed with honey and curd before use. Apply the paste and leave it on for 20 minutes. If sour curd is used, it helps to make the skin fairer.

Mix together one egg and one cup masoor dal. Dry in the sun for 3 days. Dry 100 gm neem leaves in the shade. Powder together. Store in a jar. Mix with honey and curd before use. This is essentially a high protein pack.

For oily skin, three teaspoonfuls multani mitti, three tsps with hazel, five drops eau de cologne, half tsp rose water. Make a paste and apply on the face and neck. Wash off after 20 minutes. Three tablespoonsful oatmeal, three tbsp witch hazel, half tsp glycerine. Mix together and apply over face and neck. Wash off after 20 minutes.

For dry skin. Take juice of three plums, three strawberries and a piece of beetroot. Mix in sandalwood powder. Apply over face and neck. Wash off after 20 minutes. Two tbsp oatmeal, one tsp olive oil, half tsp fresh cream. Mix together and apply over face and neck. Wash off after 20 minutes.

Facial

Indulge in a facial once a month but only if your skin is pimple-free. Try this right in your home. Tie the hair back. Cleanse face with freshly skimmed-milk for oily skin and whole for dry skin. Mix a little fresh cream and haldi. Massage into face and neck in upward and outward movements from chin to the temples. Continue for 15 minutes. Steam face. Press out blackheads if any. Give yourself a face pack-whichever you choose. Wash off after dry. If old pimple marks are present, rub the rice pack mentioned earlier. Conclude with a cold compress—a handkerchief dipped in ice-cold water pressed against the face.

These are only a few beauty hints based on kitchen ingredients of daily use. Mundane as they are, they are easily available and inexpensive. And surprisingly enough, they work—just as well as they did in the good old days! The next time we encounter the ordinary cucumber or the homely cauliflower, we may perhaps accord our daily kitchen companions a little more respect than we have been so far! Below are some more age-old home cosmetics:

Feet

Cracks in the feet are not a pretty sight. Soak your feet in warm water, containing radish leaves, salt and epsom salt. If radish leaves are not available, spinach leaves can be used. The epsom salt gives your relief from aches and pains. Soaking your feet in the warm water softens the skin on the feet, making it easier to scrape off the dead skin with a pumice stone or a scraper. Apply any medicated cream or vaseline and rub into the cracks, wear socks and keep your feet raised on a stool as often in the day as you can since cracks occur only due to bad blood circulation. If your feet have black marks, shoe-bites or black ankles, rub lime juice into your feet fifteen minutes before your bath.

Hands

Brittle nails can be checked by soaking them in 1 cup of water with 1 tsp gelatine. Dry your hands and massage them with fresh cream. For dark knuckles and elbows, use lime juice or a mixture of glycerine, rose water and lime juice. Rough hands can be softened with a paste of multani mitti, malai and honey. If the roughness is around the nails, cap finger tips with the paste. Leave on for 20 minutes and wash off with cold water. Rough hands can be treated with a mixture of glycerine, rose water and almond oil to soften them.

Removing Hair

You can now wax off unwanted hair right at home. It is so simple to make the wax at home if you have the ingredients and the inclination. Take 3 cups of sugar, 1 cup lime juice. Heat on low fire stirring all the time. When the sugar dissolves completely, the colour will change. Put a drop of this mixture into a cup of water. It must not settle to the bottom in a bead form nor should it dissolve. When it settles to the bottom in a flat form, it is ready for use. Apply the wax in the direction of the growth of the hair. Press a strip of cloth over it. Pull off in one stroke.

Beauty Aids

For a peaches-and cream complexion, prepare at home time-tested money-saving, effective beauty aids from fruits and vegetables to maintain a flawless complexion and a soft, lovely radiance.

Astringent Lotion

Extract juice from a small apricot. To this add one-fourth teaspoon each of lime and tomato juice. Mix well. Spread the lotion over your face and neck. Leave it on for about fifteen minutes. It serves as a very good astringent. Wash off with lukewarm water and splash on some cold water.

Tomato Lotion

Add a couple of drops of lime juice to a tablespoon of tomato juice. Mix well before applying the lotion over your face. Leave it on for half an hour before removing with ordinary tap water. This lotion takes care of enlarged pores, shrinking them effectively.

Water Lemon Lotion

Squeeze out juice of a small piece of water melon. Apply it over your face. Leave it on for fifteen minutes before washing it off with warm water and splashing cold water. This lotion freshens up the skin and clears it of all the blemishes.

Orange Tonic

Grind and make a paste of two kernels of almonds. Stir in one tablespoonful each of orange and carrot juice and two tablespoonfuls, of milk. Mix well. Apply the tonic to your face and neck. Let it remain for an hour or so. Wash it off with water. Its regular use will improve scars left by chicken pox if the treatment starts immediately after recovery from the disease.

Radish Lotion

Extract juice from a small piece of radish. Add to it equal quantity of buttermilk. Stir well. Apply the lotion over your face. Wash it off one hour after application with hot water and then splash on some cold water on your face. It is an excellent lotion for counteracting freckles.

Whitening Lotion

Stir in a dash of turmeric powder and lime juice one tablespoonful of cucumber juice. Mix well and apply over your face and neck. Leave it on for half an hour. Then wash it off with ordinary tap water. It is an excellent whitener for all types of skin.

Cleansing Lotion

Stir in one teaspoonful each of cucumber juice and milk a quarter teaspoonful of lime juice. Mix well and apply over your face and neck. Leave it on for fifteen minutes and wash off with lukewarm water and splash on some cold water. This lotion will clanse the pores of the skin.

Bleaching Lotion

Stir in half a teaspoonful of honey and a few drops of milk a teaspoonful of lime juice. Mix well and apply over your face and neck fifteen minutes before taking bath. This lotion has mild bleaching action on greasy skin.

Cucumber Tonic

Squeeze out juice from a small cucumber. Add to it one-fourth teaspoonful each of rose water and lime juice. Stir well. Apply over your face and neck. Leave it on for fifteen minutes before washing off with lukewarm water and splash on some cold water. Good for a dull and greasy complexion.

Cabbage Mask

Squeeze juice from two cabbage leaves. Dissolve in it five gm of yeast and stir in one teaspoonful of honey. Mix well and apply thickly over your face and neck. Leave it on for fifteen minutes. Remove it with a cottonwool soaked in water. This lotion will counteract any tendency to wrinkles and dryness, giving complexion a rose-petal softness.

Mint Lotion

Extract juice from a handful of mint leaves. Before retiring at night apply the juice over your face. In the morning wash your face with water. This lotion eases away pimples and blemishes at the same time leaving your skin soft and smooth.

Inner Beauty

Women spend a fortune on clothes and other accessories. A great chunk of one's shopping time is taken over in hunting for the right shade of lipstick or the right brand of mascara.

True, all these things give a fillip to one's appearance; but how many of us realise how important that 'internal glow'—the result of inner harmony—is to our looks?

No shade of lipstick beautifies the lips as effectively as a spontaneous smile; no mascara or eyeliner can do such wonders to your eyes as does that spark of cheerfulness!

Stress and negative thoughts are the main enemies of beauty. Half the battle is won if they are kept under check! The best remedy for these maladies is, of course, relaxation. For most, it just means leaving all work and resting on the bed or armchair; for others the term brings to mind cool hill resorts and a long holiday.

But any pleasant deviation from the routine itself is relaxation, and it is this, that we have to practise.

Break Monotony

Never set a rigid schedule for this period but carry on with whatever you feel like doing. To make this time more interesting, rotate your activities. If you paint one day, read a good book on the second and just sit and watch the beauty of nature around you on the third!

If you are too busy a housewife and are not able to spare even this much of time for yourself, why not then squeeze out a few minutes in between your daily routine for the same? Why not leaf through the pages of your favourite magazine while the cooker is cooking the daal for lunch?

Or, take time off to inspect your new pot plant while your bath water is being heated.

These small pleasures of life are far more relaxing than, perhaps, attending parties in overcrowded hotels, watching a movie in a stuffy theatre, or looking at the idiot box (TV) for hours on end.

Taking up work requiring physical effort and concentration, is another good way of overcoming stress and tension. People without any hobbies, whatsoever, are very rare.

Further the interests and talents you are adept at, and see how it reduces your tension and stress, apart from giving your pleasure.

Develop Hobbies

According to your ability, create something which you can call your own, something you can be proud of, something which gives you a tremendous sense of achievement—whether it be a tasty dish or an intricate piece of embroidery.

This is an era of action, and though it sounds a contradiction in terms, keeping active itself is, in a sense, relaxation. Studies have shown that depression is common to students during vacation times, when they have nothing to do.

Reserve a place for yourself in the kitchen or elsewhere with a comfortable chair or a folding cot, for you to relax with a book or knitting when time permits. Short periods of relaxation in between work are more beneficial than long stretches of illness.

When you are doing monotonous jobs, switch on your transistor or put on your favourite number on the cassette player, for music is one of the best soothers of the mind.

Bottling up feelings is harmful and leads to more stress and related problems. Any problem can be talked over with a good friend, or with yourself; it gives instant relief.

A good memory is a wonderful thing but there are times when it is more important to forget! If we are to enjoy good health, there may be some things which are best forgotten instead of being left to fester, with harmful emotions in our minds.

Pets

Pets are also good 'shock absorbers' and tension-relievers. Apart from giving one a tremendous sense of responsibility, they heal one's bruised ego.

An American expert says, 'Certain social conventions prevent people from touching one another. Animals are a means of expressing this need-a way of getting that kind of comfort.

'There are sometimes boring and personal things which we want to pour out. Pets come to our aid as patient, quiet and probably interesting listeners.'

Relaxation Techniques

There is a great release of tension after sharing a guilt feeling or problem with a pet. Tests have revealed that tension levels are at their lowest when pets are around!

This is the age of yoga and even westerners are finding solace in it. There is no tranquilliser as effective as the 'shavasana', the yogic exercise done in the pose of a shava or a dead body. Even amateurs can practise it.

Lie on your back (without a pillow), with your arms and legs straight and a little away from your body.

Close your eyes, push all other thoughts away from your mind and visualise each of your limbs going limp and lifeless-starting from your toes and feet and ending at your forehead and head.

Then repeat it the other way round, starting from your head downwards. Breathe deeply, and relax for another 10 to 15 minutes, with your eyes closed, and concentrate on your breathing alone.

Releasing in a tub of warm water is also beneficial, for warm water is very soothing. If you don't have a tub, take a leisurely bath daily, and at times, take time off for an oil massage and bath-grandma's good old recipe for beauty and muscular rejuvenation.

Massage your head and body well with a bath oil or any other warm oil of your choice and take a relaxing bath in warm water and watch your tension being washed away!

Shun Negativity

Checking negative feelings, like hate, jealousy, anger, etc., is also within your own interests because these are going to neither benefit you nor others around you.

A mature person should open up his or her heart to the joys and sorrows of others, rejoicing in their achievements and grieving in their losses.

Only this type of involvement gives one a sense of belonging to the world around, which, in turn, gives a purpose to life and helps to check negative feelings to a very great extent.

All these are just means to an end. In the final analysis, it requires your determined effort to achieve a cool mentality which is the real secret of beauty.

This 'cosmetic' suits all skin types and is free of cost. It is rightly said, 'It requires 62 muscles to frown, while only 38 are required for smiling.'

Drink More Water—Shed More Fat

Doctors and nutritionists swear by the formula, and parents faithfully hand it down to their children (whether or not they abide by it themselves): eight glasses of water a day. They talk about its health-giving properties (how good it is for your skin and your system, how it flushes away toxins and wastes, how it aids digestion and relieves constipation). But, has any doctor told you about how water can flush away the fat?

Flush away the fat? Come again.

Yes, it's incredible, but it's true. At least, according to top diet doctor, Donalt S. Robertson, author of a book on the subject, **'The Snowbird Diet.'**

His recommendations are bolstered by studies in the West that are increasingly indicating that when water intake drops, fat deposits go up. And the even more interesting converse—an increased water intake can actually reduce fat deposits.

How's that? Here's how (it's that bad old vicious cycle at work). When you don't drink enough water, your kidneys can't function properly. As a consequence, they dump some of their work-load on to the liver.

When the liver is landed with some of the kidney's functions, it cannot work to full capacity on its own job. And, one of the primary functions of the liver is to metabolize stored fat into energy. When it's working below par, the liver metabolizes less fat, so that some of it remains stored up in the body, resulting in weight gain or, at best, inhibiting weight loss.

That's not the only way in which water is related to obesity: Paradoxically, the problem of oedema (fluid retention in the body) is often caused by too little water intake. This is what happens: When your water intake is too little, the body alerts its mechanisms to what it sees as a potential 'survival threat.'

In a defensive reaction, it begins to grasp at whatever is available, holding onto every last drop that it gets. This water is then stored in extracellular spaces (outside the cells) and manifests itself as oedemas (swollen feet, legs and hands).

If you have a chronic problem of fluid retention, it could also be caused by excess of salts in the body. The more salts, the more the water retained by the body to dilute them.

Water is also an important adjunct to any weight loss programme. It helps to combat the sagging skin phenomenon that occurs during weight reduction—by literally buoying up the shrinking cells and 'plumping' out the skin, leaving it clear and fresh. Similarly, it keeps the muscles well-toned and firmed up, giving them their natural ability to contract.

Besides, when you are dieting, you have to be careful to avoid dehydration, and drinking lots of water can help to maintain the fluid balance in the body.

Also, during weight loss, the body has to offload a much larger amount of metabolized fat. A correspondingly larger intake of water is needed to shed this waste.

Conversely, it follows that overweight people (with larger metabolic loads to convert into energy) need more water to prod along the metabolism.

Experts point to water's ability to suppress the appetite naturally. "Drinking water creates a sense of fullness. Anyone who has a glass of water before a meal, is bound to eat less, so there is a natural diet control at work here."

How much water should you drink? The eight-glasses-a-day maxim largely holds good, but according to Dr. Robertson, the overweight person needs one additional glass for every 25 pounds of excess weight. The intake would also vary according to other factors. So, if you do brisk exercise, you naturally drink more water. In a tropical climate like ours, one should have a glass of water every two hours—which works out to about 8/10 glasses a day.

Even drinking a little more cannot harm your body. The excess is simply secreted in urine or sweat. More than 90 percent of a child's weight, and over 50 per cent of an adult's, is made up of the water constituent in the body. So, you really need a lot of water during the day to make up the loss from perspiration, exhalation and urination. 'Never ignore a thirst', say the experts, 'It is the best guide to your body's needs.'

Of course, many other beverages contain water, as do many foods—but you just can't beat the natural goodness of plain, pure water. It's the best thirst quencher of all, because it's devoid of harmful additives and, of course, is non-fattening!

Should you avoid water during meals? That's another maxim that's generously handed around, but according to experts there is really no evidence to support the claim that drinking water during meals is in any way harmful to the body. In fact, water is known to aid digestion—only, too much of it during meals can dilute the digestive enzymes.

Apart from its catalyst action in weight reduction, water is also one of the most basic of beauty aids. Drinking plenty of water will literally alter your appearance, bringing a natural glow to your skin and a sparkle to your eyes. No moisturizer or eye-drops can do as much!

Water should preferably be drunk cold, says Dr. Robertson. It is absorbed more quickly by the body than warm water. And getting back to its role in weight loss, he adds that there is some evidence to suggest that drinking cold water can actually help to burn up calories!

So, cut down on the colas and the camparis. You've nothing to lose but your flab.

Make Your Own Herbal Cosmetics

Making cosmetics at home does not involve great chemical knowledge or extra-special equipment.

The recipes given below are basically for 'hygienic' cosmetics rather than 'aesthetic' ones—which means that they are also suitable for men-after all they too wash their hair, take baths and have need of dusting powders, deodorants, skin lotions and creams.

Basically you will need:

1. Enamel bowl
2. Measuring spoons
3. A set of measuring cups
4. An electric beater
5. A good strong sieve
6. An eye dropper
7. Jars and bottles.

Now here are the recipes starting with the hair down to your feet.

For the Hair

1. **Herbal Shampoo**

   100 gm Reetha (soap nuts)

   50 gm Shikakai

   50 gm Amla

   Soak all these ingredients at night in 2 glasses of water for 12 hours. Then boil till it is reduced to ½ glass. When cool squeeze it nicely and then strain.

2. **Rich Protein Pack**

   1 whole egg, juice of half a lime

   Egg protein is excellent for the hair. Beat the egg and lime juice and apply on the hair. Leave on for an hour. This pack is very good for dandruff too.

3. **Deep Conditioning Henna Pack**

   1 cup henna powder

   Juice of one lemon

   A small piece of katta (powdered)

   1 tbsp coffee powder

   1 egg

   tea water (enough to make a paste)

   curd (optional)

   Mix all the ingredients and leave overnight. Apply on hair the next morning and keep on for an hour or two for glossy hair. Omit the curd if you want to get the henna colour.

4. **For Black Hair**

   Ingredients are the same as for henna mixture except curd. Add amla powder. Heat the amla powder in an iron kadai. Mix it with the henna mixture and leave overnight in the kadai. Apply on the hair the next morning and keep for an hour or two.

5. **A Fresh Herbal Shine Pack**

   Leaves of hibiscus, tulsi, mint, marigold, neem, bael an balsam.

   Grind these leaves to a fine paste. The hibiscus leaves will make it sticky. Apply on hair and keep for two hours. Wash off with a mild shampoo.

6. **Floral Shampoo**

   1 tablespoonful of flowers or herbs

   1½ tablespoonfuls borax

   1½ tablespoonfuls sodium sesquicarbonate

   2 tablespoonfuls flaked soap

Carefully combine the ingredients with a pestle and mortar. To use, dissolve 2 tablespoonfuls of the powder in 3 fluid oz. of hot water, leave to soak for a few minutes—till cool enough to use.

7. **Lemon Shampoo**

   1 oz lemon balm leaves

   1 pint boiling water

   2 tablespoonfuls sodium sesquicarbonate

   5 tablespoonfuls of flaked soap

   a few drops of oil of lemons

   With half a pint of boiling water make an infusion of the lemon balm; in the other half melt the sodium sesquicarbonate and the flaked soap. Strain the infusion and combine both liquids, adding the oil of lemons. Use about a cupful of shampoo for your hair.

Conditioners

If you have dry or brittle hair, any of the vegetable oils can act as a marvellous conditioner.

8. **Oil Conditioner**

   2 tablespoonfuls vegetable oil

   Slowly heat the oil in a double saucepan. When warmed massage it onto your scalp and then all through your hair; cover the whole of your head with a plastic shower hat (a polythene bag will do just as well). Cover that, turban fashion, with a well warmed towel (the quickest way is to soak it in hot water and wring out the surplus). When the towel becomes cold, repeat once again, then shampoo your hair as usual making sure you remove all excess oil.

9. **Rich Hair Conditioner**

   1 egg

   1 teaspoonful honey

   2 teaspoonfuls vegetable oil

   Combine the ingredients in a double saucepan and massage, steam and shampoo as before.

10. **Mild Hair Conditioner**

Whisk an egg until fluffy and rub it into your scalp, leave on for about 5 minutes and rinse off with tepid warm water before shampooing. Don't use hot water or you may get a headful of scrambled egg!

11. **Herbal Vinegar Rinse for Dandruff and Excess Oil**

¼ pint herbal vinegar or apple vinegar

2 pints water

Mix the vinegar with the water and use this solution as a final rinse after shampooing.

12. **Hair Oil for Falling Hair**

1 kg coconut oil, 6 orange peels (fresh or dried)

100 gm amla

500 gm Naag Kesar or 100 gm shikakai

50 gms methi seeds

Put all these ingredients (except methi seeds) in the oil and soak overnight. Next day boil the oil till the peels turn black. The oil should not smoke.Cool and add the methi seeds. Strain after 8 days.

13. **Dandruff Oil**

Take the same prepared oil and add 2 tsp of Arniflour Ayurvedic oil for 1 kg.

14. **Hair Dyes and Colourants**

Probably the oldest hair colouring agent is henna. It is almost impossible to predict the exact colour change that will take place as the original colour and condition of the hair, and the length of time the powder is left on, play such an important part. The only way to get a vague idea is to do a 'test' before embarking on what might be an irrevocable step.

15. **Henna Powder Hair Dye**

Put some powder in a bowl and to it add enough hot water to make a paste. Wet your hair and with a brush completely cover all your hair or the parts to be coloured with the paste. Cover your head with tin foil or a plastic bag until you think your hair is coloured sufficiently. Test by cleaning a few strands of hair to see that colour change has taken place. The process can be speeded up if you dry the paste with a hair dryer. When completed wash the paste off with warm water and shampoo as usual.

16. **Walnut Brown Hair Dye**

6 tablespoonfuls green walnut skins

1-3/4 tablespoonfuls alum powder

3-1/2 fl. oz. orange flower water

Finely chop up the walnut skins and mix to a paste with the alum and orange flower water. Put the paste on to your hair and leave for about an hour, rinse off with warm water and shampoo as usual.

Grey hair can have a lot of its original colour restored if you rinse it with a strong infusion of sage leaves, or mix the infusion to a paste with kaolin powder and proceed as before.

17. **Setting Lotions**

If you have either limp bodiless hair or straight hair that could do with a bit of bounce, try rinsing it with beer (doesn't matter if it's flat) after a shampoo. It works very well and you won't smell like a brewery either! Lemon juice too works well as a setting lotion, but preferably on light or very greasy hair. Strain the juice of a freshly squeezed lemon and comb it into the hair and set as usual.

18. **To Soothe Tired Eyes**

Make a mild infusion of parsley, chamomile, fennel (saunf) and when tepid, use as an eye wash.

Squeeze the juice from ¼ of a cucumber and use that as an eye bath or place a slice of it over each closed eye.

Ordinary cold tea can be used to good advantage as an eye lotion and especially soothing are two tea bags dipped in cold water until the leaves have expanded: squeeze out the excess water and put over each closed eye, put your feet up and relax for ten minutes.

19. **To Reduce Puffiness**

Grate a raw potato and put a teaspoonful on two small squares of muslin to cover each closed eye. Put your feet up and leave these compresses on for about ¼ hour and then splash with cold water.

20. **Eye make-up Remover**

2 tablespoonfuls almond oil

1 tablespoonful castor oil

Mix the two oils, soak a piece of cotton wool in it and gently wipe away any eye make-up.

For Teeth, Mouth and Lips

21. **Tooth Cleaning Pastes**

A very effective but far from attractive paste can be made by crushing some charred bread to a fine powder and mixing it with a few drops of peppermint oil.

Should you have any doubts as to the freshness and sweetness of your breath, try using a decoction of corn flowers or an infusion of mint as a mouthwash, or even rosewater. Sometimes, chewing a couple of cloves or a sprig or two of parsley is effective in purifying the breath.

22. **Breath-fresh Pastilles**

¼ oz. lavender flowers

3/4 oz. icing sugar

enough egg white to bind together.

Blend the ingredients together until quite smooth and roll into little balls, leave in a dry place till set firm.

23. **Lip Gloss**

2 tablespoonfuls cocoa butter

½ teaspoonful beewax

Melt the wax and combine with the cocoa butter. Pour into a pot ready for use. Apply with a lip brush.

For the Face

The best soaps to use as facial cleansers are rich, nourishing ones that will not leave the skin over-dry. Work up a lather using warm water and a soft nylon complexion brush. Spread it over your face, avoiding the eyes and the delicate skin around them, using a circular movement and paying special attention to the area around your nose. Rinse the lather off with warm water and pat dry with a soft towel, followed by a mild toning lotion or cream.

Oatmeal too can be a very effective cleanser both for face and body.

24. **Oatmeal Cleanser**

2 oz. oatmeal

3-4 tablespoonfuls milk

Grind the oatmeal to a fine powder, warm the milk and add it to the oatmeal to form a paste. Use this as a facial scrub using a complexion brush as before (a particularly good way of removing dead cells and deep cleaning the pores) and wash off with warm water.

25. **Curd and Lemon Cleansing Milk**

1 tablespoonful natural curd

1 teaspoonful lemon juice

Mix the curd and the lemon juice and apply to the face with cotton wool. Clean off with tissue.

26. **Mild Cleansing Milk**

¼ pint milk

¼ cucumber

Squeeze the juice from the cucumber and mix it with the milk. Apply to your face with cotton wool and wipe excess off with tissue.

27. **Apple Cleansing Lotion**

1 big apple

1 tablespoonful milk

1 tablespoonful fuller's earth powder

Squeeze the juice from the apple and combine it with the milk and powder.

28. **Simple, No-effort Cleansers**

Fresh potato juice or strawberry juice

Warmed milk, natural yogurt

Any of the vegetable oils.

Cleansing Cream

29. **Basic Light Cleansing Cream**

½ oz. beewax

3 fl oz. almond oil

¼ teaspoonful borax

2½ fl. oz. distilled water

Slowly melt the wax with the almond oil in a double saucepan. Dissolve the borax in the warmed water (do make sure it really has dissolved otherwise the cream will be lumpy). Add the borax solution to the wax and oil. Remove the pan from the heat and stir until cool or beat with a whisk until it thickens and becomes creamy.

30. **Rich Avacodo Cleansing Cream**

½ oz. beewax

1 oz. lanolin

3 fl. oz avocado oil

2½ fl. oz. distilled water

In a double saucepan, melt the lanolin and wax and add the oil. When combined, remove the pan from the heat and slowly stir in the water. Stir or whisk until the cream is quite cool.

In both these recipes you can substitute a herbal infusion of your choice instead of the distilled water, or add a few drops of essential oil, then add perfume. The vegetable oils too are interchangeable.

31. **Mayonnaise Cleansing Cream**

1 egg

¼ pint olive oil

1 tablespoonful cider vinegar

½ teaspoonful sugar

Blend the egg, vinegar and sugar and slowly add the oil, beating all the time, until the mixture thickens and turns golden yellow.

32. **Cleansing Jelly**

1 tsp. gelatine

2 tsp honey

¼ cup glycerine

½ tsp alcohol

2 tbsp water

Soak the gelatine in water. Place in a double boiler and dissolve over low heat. Remove from heat and when lukewarm add remaining ingredients.

33. **Rose Cleansing Cream**

½ tsp lanolin

1 tbsp petroleum jelly

4 tbsp mineral oil

10 tbsp water

5 drops rose extract

Melt all the ingredients except water. Add warm water to it and keep stirring continuously. Remove from heat and continue to beat together till cool.

34. **Cucumber Cleansing Cream**

3 tsp white wax

4 tsp coconut oil

5 tsp olive oil

4 tbsp cucumber juice

1 tsp glycerine

1 pinch of borax

Melt the wax and oils over the pan of boiling water. Simultaneously heat the cucumber juice, glycerine and borax in a separate bowl, till the borax has dissolved completely. When the contents of both bowls are melted, mix them, and add water drop by drop stirring continuously. Remove it from heat and beat until the mixture is thick and cool. Store the cream in the refrigerator.

35. **Steam Cleansing**

The deepest cleansing treatment is steam, though we do not advise it if your skin is at all sensitive or you have breathing difficulties.

Add a tablespoonful of herbs to a pint of boiling water in a large bowl. Hold your face about 12 inches above the bowl and drape a towel over your head and the bowel rim. Steam your face for about 5 minutes. After steaming, wipe with cotton wool or tissue to remove impurities and close the pores by splashing with cold water or a herbal infusion. For the total face treatment leave the pores open and apply a face mask followed by herbal infusion.

Traditionally, limeflowers and chamomile flowers have been used as steam facial herbs, but you can experiment with any herbs you like either singly or combined. Those to be recommended are peppermint, basil, marigold nasturtium, fennel, thyme, lady's mantel, nettle, yarrow, houseleek and comfrey.

36. **Face Masks**

Face masks are more effective in cleansing and toning the skin if applied when the pores are open. If you cannot take the steam treatment, try dipping a face cloth into hot water, wringing out the surplus and covering your face with the cloth for a few minutes before applying a mask. Using a mask also can act as a general 'pick-me-up' because for them to have a chance to 'set' you really need to relax completely with your feet up-normally about 15 minutes—a good opportunity too for refreshing your eyes with a cool compress.

Almost any herbs, fruits and vegetables can be used in a face mask, either alone, mixed or combined with thickeners such as buttermilk, cream, curd, honey, egg, fuller's earth, kaolin powder or oatmeal. Basically what you do is chop a couple of handfuls of herbs and simmer for about 10 minutes in a pan containing either milk or water (enough to prevent them from burning); or mash whatever fruit or vegetables you want to use. If the mixture is particularly runny, thicken it, and cover your face with it. If the idea of actual pieces of vegetation on your face does not appeal, extract the juices and use those instead. Leave the mask on until 'set' and wash off with warm water, finally splashing with cold water, and preferably dabbing on a tonic or an astringent lotion to close the pores.

37. **Herbs, Fruits, Vegetables and other Material for Face Masks**

Paresley

Plain egg white beaten till almost stiff

Honey mixed with egg yolk and a teaspoonful of oil

Mashed cucumber mixed with yogurt and kaolin powder

Thick cream mixed with honey

Mashed tomato and oatmeal

Carrot and curd

Avocado mixed with honey and lemon juice

Powdered yeast mixed with yogurt and kaolin powder

Orange juice and honey mixed with buttermilk and oatmeal
Lettuce and curd

There are hundreds of variations to the face mask theme so it is just a question of trying anything you like the sound of—or inventing your own.

38. **Astringent Lotions and Skin Tonics**

Astringent lotions will close the pores of the skin after a face mask, and also help in reducing blackheads and blemishes in general by removing excess oils. Strong lotions usually contain alcohol in some form and should only be used occasionally on particularly greasy skin.

The milder lotions and tonics are basically herbal and can be splashed or patted on to the skin more freely and regularly.

Find a small basin and cut several pieces of thick lint or gauze to fit neatly inside it, and soak them in one of the lotions. You will then always have a useful pot of handy 'freshener' pads with which to wipe your face. Any surplus lotion could be wiped off with a tissue. Particularly useful for wiping the face after using a cleansing cream.

39. **Herbal Vinegar Astringent Lotion**

1 tablespoonful herbal vinegar

¼ pint distilled water

Pour into a bottle, shake to combine.

40. **Almond Astringent**

2 teaspoonfuls ground almonds

1 teaspoonful borax

1½ teaspoonfuls tincture of benzoin

½ pint rosewater

2½ fl. oz. distilled water

Dissolve the borax in the tincture and add the rosewater to it. Blend the almonds with the distilled water and pour all of it into a bottle. Shake to blend and label it before using.

41. **Vinegar Astringent**

½ cup vinegar

¼ cup water

3 tbsp rose water

Mix the liquids and bottle.

42. **Neem Tonic**

5-6 neem leaves

2 cups water

Boil the leaves in water. Cool and strain the liquid.

43. **Lemon Astringent**

3 tbsp lemon juice

1 cup rose water

Mix the liquids and bottle.

44. **Mild Astringents**

These are basically herbal infusions which do not contain any spirits.

Parsley, fennel, have light astringent properties; they are useful if your skin needs a gentler clean.

Herbal Anti-wrinkle Lotions

Stress, aging, faulty diet and improper rest contribute towards the formation of wrinkles and stress lines on the face. Regular massaging, facial exercises and the application of anti-wrinkle creams can forestall the appearance of wrinkles. Herbal anti-wrinkle lotions are soothing and gentle.

45. **Multi Anti-wrinkle Lotion**

    2 tbsp mint mixture

    4 drops peppermint extract

    a pinch of alum powder

    Mix the ingredients thoroughly and store in a glass jar.

46. **Cucumber Anti-wrinkle Lotion**

    1 egg white

    1 tsp lemon juice

    1 tsp vodka or alcohol

    ¼ cucumber mashed and seived

    Extract juice from the mashed cucumber. Beat the egg white. Mix the juice with the rest of the ingredients.

47 (a) **Pimple Pack**

1 tsp Gopichand powder

½ teaspoonful camphor

¼ teaspoonful alum

Mix with rosewater and apply only for pimple skin.

47 (b) **Pimple Sear Pack**

100 gm Neem (fresh or dry)

100 gm Tulsi

100 gm mint

Grind all these together, make a paste with milk and apply.

Herbal Nourishing Creams

If you are over 30 or if you have dry and flaky skin, you need to moisturise and cream your face daily. Nourishment helps restore natural oils.

48. **Almond Cream**

4 tbsp lanolin

3 tbsp almond oil

2 tbsp rose water

Put the lanolin and almond oil in a glass bowl. Place the bowl in a pan of hot water and heat over a low flame, stirring continuously until the contents of the bowl melt to a smooth paste. Remove the bowl from the hot water and add rose water to it. Mix well.

49. **Lanolin Night Cream**

6 tbsp glycerine

6 tbsp lanolin

6 tbsp rose water

Melt the ingredients in a bowl placed in hot water. Beat well and cool.

50. **Avacado Nourishing Cream**

1 teaspoonful beeswax

pinch of borax

1 tablespoonful almond oil

3 tablespoonfuls avocado oil

1 tablespoonful rosewater

Melt the oils and the wax in a double saucepan. Dissolve the borax in the rosewater and add to the oils, stirring until cool, rich and creamy.

51. **Simple Nourishing Cream**

2 teaspoonfuls honey

1 egg white

few drops of almond oil

Beat the egg white and add it to the honey; stir in the oil of almonds.

52. **Moisturising Cream**

1 teaspoonful beeswax

pinch of borax

½ teaspoonful vegetable margarine or cocoa butter

2½ teaspoonfuls coconut oil

2 tablespoonfuls distilled water

½ teaspoonful lanolin

Melt the wax, margarine, oil and lanolin in a double saucepan. Dissolve the borax in the warmed water and add it to the oils, beating until the mixture cools. (Odourless coconut oil should be used).

53. **Honey Night Cream**

3 tbsp lanolin

½ tbsp honey

Put honey and lanolin in a bowl and place it in hot water till it melts. Slowly add 4 tbsp warm water to it, beating continuously until it cools.

53 (a) **Cucumber Moisturising Cream**

2 tablespoonfuls cucumber juice

1 teaspoonful lanolin

½ teaspoonful cocoa butter

2½ teaspoonfuls coconut oil

pinch of borax

1 teaspoonful beeswax

Proceed as for previous cream. Combine the juice and borax and beat them into the oils.

54. **Lettuce Moisturising Lotion**

1 lettuce

½ pint distilled water

Boil the lettuce leaves in the water for about 10 minutes. Leave till cool, then strain and bottle.

55. **Herbal Dairy Cream**

2 tablespoonfuls double cream

1 tablespoonful herb juice

Beat together until thick and pot up for use.

56. **Rosewater Moisture Lotion**

4 tablespoonfuls glycerine

3 tablespoonfuls rosewater

Pour into a bottle and shake before use.

For the Body

Bathing

Taking a bath can be turned into a luxurious and deliciously scented event with the help of a few well chosen soaps, herbs and oils.

The most usual cleansing ingredient in taking a bath, apart from hot water, is a cake of a soap and there are several ways of making them at home without using animal fats or tallow.

Before you start making your own soap, a few words of warning: Be very careful when using caustic soda-if even a speck of it gets on to your skin, wash immediately with cold water, lemon juice or vinegar or you may get a horribly painful burn. Always wear rubber gloves to avoid this.

Try not to breathe the fumes from the soda when mixing it with the water or the oils—it could damage your lungs!

Never use aluminium, tin, or foil containers, because the soda will gradually eat its way through amidst frothy evil smelling bubbles!

Bearing these words of caution in mind making soap is quite straightforward.

57. **Rich Complexion Soap**

2 tablespoonfuls caustic soda

7½ fl. oz. water

10 fl. oz almond oil

4 oz. coconut oil

2 teaspoonfuls glycerine or honey

Put the water into a glass or ceramic bowl and, wearing rubber gloves, carefully measure the caustic soda and slowly stir it into the water using a wooden spoon, until dissolved. Melt the coconut and almond oils with the glycerine in an enamel saucepan until warm. The soda solution will have got quite hot so leave it until just warm before pouring it slowly, while stirring into the oils. Keep stirring until the mixture thickens (this could take upto 15 minutes, so do persevere). If the mixture congeals just place the saucepan in a basin of hot water and stir it till it gets back to a good pouring consistency.

Line three plastic or wooden boxes, about 2½ " x 3" and 1" deep, with pieces of polythene (to help lift the hardened soap from the moulds) and pour the thickened mixture into them. Put the boxes on a tray, cover with a piece of cardboard, wrap in a towel or blanket and put it in a warm dry place until set (This should happen in 24 hours but sometimes it takes longer). When set, lift the soap from the moulds, peel off the polythene, wrap it in greaseproof paper and store in a cool dry place until quite hard (at least two weeks). This makes a lovely pure white soap.

58. **Simple Bath Soap**

4 heaped tablespoonfuls caustic soda

½ pint water

2 tablespoonfuls olive oil

2 tablespoonfuls coconut oil

2 tablespoonfuls vegetable margarine

Proceed exactly as before substituting the margarine for the glycerine or honey.

If you want to add colour, perfume or nourishing ingredients to your simple soap do so just before pouring the thickened liquid into the moulds for setting, and combine thoroughly by stirring. Add a few drops of any essential oils-only two at a time and stir thoroughly-too strong a smell will be off-putting. Try adding a couple of spoonfuls of mashed avocado, strawberry, cucumber, oatmeal, Irish moss, ground almonds, chopped fresh herbs or flowers and a little colouring either to match your bathroom decor or echo the natural colour of the extra ingredients or perfume. Try carving the soaps into shapes or engraving your initials into it before you wrap it up to finally harden.

If the idea of using caustic soda frightens you, try making a soap substitute.

59. **Almond Soap Substitute**

2 tablespoonfuls finely ground almonds

2 tablespoonfuls kaolin powder

½ teaspoonful borax

few drops oil of almonds

Mix all ingredients together and use a knob of it instead of soap.

Body Lotions and Tonics

After bathing you may like to tone up your skin by splashing with a cool lotion. The simplest tonic is cold water—but you could use rosewater, elderflower water, any cold herbal infusions, cologne, floral water or herbal vinegars, diluted one part vinegar to eight parts water.

60. **Rose and Lime Body Lotion**

3 tablespoonfuls rose water

1 tablespoonful glycerine

2 tablespoonful lime juice

Mix the ingredients and store in a glass bottle.

For Hands and Nails

Nails

To strengthen finger nails

Rub pure lanolin into cuticles each night.

Paint nails with white iodine after each immersion into water.

Mix equal parts of castor oil and glycerine and rub into fingertips and cuticles.

Soak fingertips in a strong infusion of dill.

To colour finger nails:

Make a thick paste with henna powder and warm water.

Leave on until quite dry, then wash off paste. The nails will then have a pinky tinge to them.

Hand Care

61. **Almond Hand Cream**

2 oz. ground almonds

1 egg yolk

1 teaspoonful almond oil

¼ pint milk

Boil the gound almonds in the milk until it is absorbed. Stir in the beaten egg yolk and re-heat.

Cool and add the almond oil.

62. **Cocoa Hand Cream**

2 tablespoonfuls cocoa butter

2 tablespoonfuls almond oil

2 tablespoonfuls beeswax

Melt the butter and the wax in a double saucepan and stir in the oil. Bottle up for use.

63. **Lanolin Hand Cream**

3 tablespoonful glycerine

3 tablespoonfuls almond oil

3 tablespoonfuls lanolin

Mix the ingredients over a pan of hot water.

Barrier Creams

64. **Hand Barrier Cream**

1 oz. lanolin

½ oz. beeswax

32 fl. oz. mineral oil

2½ fl. oz. distilled water or herbal infusion

pinch of borax

Melt the lanolin and wax and combine with the mineral oil. Dissolve the borax in the water and stir into the wax and oil solution. Pot up when thick and cooled.

65. **Egg Paste Barrier Cream**

1 egg yolk

1 dessertspoon sunflower oil

Kaolin powder

Mix the egg yolk and the sunflower oil with enough kaolin powder to form a paste. Rub on the hands before doing heavy work.

66. **To Clean Stained Hands**

1 tablespoonful of sunflower oil mixed with

1 tablespoonful of sugar

Rub the mixture into your hands until clean and rinse off with water.

or

1 tablespoonful sesame oil mixed with

1 tablespoonful lemon juice

1 tablespoonful honey

Use as before.

Stained elbows can be cleaned most effectively by cleaning them with a halved lemon each for at least 5 minutes.

For the Feet

Foot Baths

To soothe tired or sore feet soak them in a bowl containing a couple of handful of nettle leaves, rosemary, lavender, mint or horsetail, covered in boiling water, but don't put your feet in until the water cools to a bearable temperature. Sea salt in hot water can also be very soothing.

If on a cold and miserably wet day you need warming up, a pinch of crushed mustard seed or powder added to hot water will soon make you feel cosy.

Nail Strengtheners and Nourishing Creams

These can be the same as those you use on your hands.

67. **Rough Skin Remover**

2 tablespoonfuls curd
1 dessertspoonful herbal or cider vinegar

Mix the two together and cover your feet with it, rubbing it well into the hard skinned parts. Leave on for about 10 minutes and rub it off followed by a warm water bath.

Floral Waters and Colognes

The simplest fragrances to make at home are floral waters. You just add about 15 drops of essential oil to a pint of distilled water and shake the bottle. The most versatile of these waters are, rosewater, orangeflower water and lavender water: but the possibilities are endless and are just a question of personal preference.

More complex 'smells' are produced by blending carefully measured amounts of oils with pure alcohol. If you want to try, and can't buy alcohol, use vodka instead.

Floral Waters

68. **Lavender Water**

10 drops oil of lavender
1 tablespoonful rosewater
3 tablespoonfuls vodka or alcohol.

69. **Melissa Water**

½ oz. lemon balm leaves, crushed
¼ oz. lemon peel, grated
¼ teaspoonful all spice
5 fl. oz. vodka or alcohol
7½ fl. oz. distilled water

Mix all together except the water, soak for a week and strain before adding the water.

70. **Hungary Water**

1 tablespoonful mint leaves, fresh
1 tablespoonful rosemary, fresh
2 fl. oz. vodka or alcohol
4 fl. oz. rosewater
grated peel of ½ of lemon and orange

Mix all together, pour into a bottle and soak for a week. Strain before using.

Colognes

71. 5 fl. oz. Vodka or alcohol

    4 tablespoonfuls rose petals, fresh

    2 tablespoonfuls lemon peel

    2 tablespoonfuls orange peel

    1 tablespoonful basil, fresh

    1 tablespoonful peppermint, fresh

    ½ pint boiling water.

    Soak the rose petals in the alcohol for a week. Crush all the leaves and grate the peel and soak in the hot water. Strain both liquids and combine in a bottle.

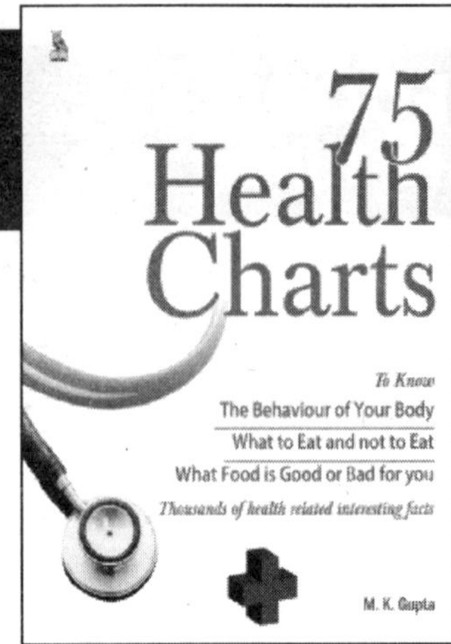

75 Health Charts

—M. K. Gupta

As any health-conscious person knows, health is truly wealth. Yet, simply harbouring good intentions does not ensure good health for anyone. Beginning in infancy and right up to our twilight years, a conscious attempt has to be made to lead a healthy lifestyle. In the formative years, our parents make this effort on our behalf. But as we enter the teens and take control of our own destinies, how well informed we are on health-related issues makes all the difference between physical well-being and ill health.

This book ensures you have all the facts, figures and data at your fingertips to promote proper health and nutrition in order to prevent disease.

In this book you will find: height and weight charts, blood pressure and pulse rate charts, calorie charts, fat and cholesterol charts, vitamin and mineral charts, balanced diet charts, pollution health hazard charts, infectious diseases and immunisation charts, healthy heart and stress charts... not to mention other relevant charts, tables and data.

So, if health has always been your problem, this book is just what the doctor ordered. And if health has been your forte, this book is exactly what the doctor would recommend to maintain you in the pink of your health. Either way, *75 Health Charts* is a must-read for all people.

Big Size • Pages: 144
Price: Rs. 120/- • Postage: Rs. 15/-